Young Children in Hospital

Based on a Memorandum written by the author and submitted to the Ministry of Health Committee on the Welfare of Sick Children in Hospital on behalf of the Tavistock Clinic and the Tavistock Institute of Human Relations.

[Young Children in Hospital]

JAMES ROBERTSON

Second Edition
with a
Postscript 1970

TAVISTOCK PUBLICATIONS

First published in 1958
by Tavistock Publications Limited
11 New Fetter Lane, London EC4P 4EE
Second Edition 1970
First published as a Social Science Paperback 1970
Reprinted twice
Reprinted 1979

ISBN 0 422 75060 3

Printed in Great Britain
at the University Press, Cambridge

CONTENTS

v

PREFACE TO THE SECOND EDITION

In 1959, a year after the publication of the first edition of this book, the Ministry of Health released its Report on *The Welfare of Children in Hospital*. In a foreword to a later publication, Sir Harry Platt, Bt., Chairman of the Committee that produced the Report, kindly acknowledged that this book and the complementary film *Going to Hospital With Mother* had had 'a strong influence' on the findings of the inquiry (120).

In the ten years following the Platt Report, many improvements have occurred in the management of children's wards, especially in the English-speaking countries, and many related publications have appeared. These deal mainly with the practical implications of a concept of care which seeks to safeguard the emotional well-being of young patients, with the responses of children and parents to better facilities, and with the problems thrown up by more enlightened paediatric practice. None of the newer publications have questioned the mental health considerations set out in the first edition.[1]

In preparing the second edition I have therefore allowed the simple statement of the first to remain unchanged. A Postscript has been added which outlines recent trends in Great Britain, with particular reference to the unique contribution of an informed public opinion mobilized to hasten the implementation of the Platt Report. Some consideration is also given to the substantial

[1] See References 60, 61, 63, 68, 79a, 82, 83, 86, 88, 90, 91, 93, 94, 95, 96, 97, 98, 99, 108, 111, 115, 116, 131, 134, 138.

Young Children in Hospital

obstacles that still stand in the way of achieving optimal care of the young child in hospital.

Tavistock Institute of Human Relations
Tavistock Centre, Belsize Lane,
London NW3

JAMES ROBERTSON
1970

PREFACE TO THE FIRST EDITION

Since 1948 The Child Development Research Unit, now sponsored jointly by the Tavistock Clinic and the Tavistock Institute of Human Relations, has been engaged in research into the effects of loss of maternal care in the early years upon the development of the total personality. As a result of this research and of a survey of the findings of other workers, the conclusion is inescapable that much emotional ill-health can be traced to disturbances in the mother-child relationship during the early years. The matter is summed up in a report for the World Health Organization, thus:

'It is essential for mental health that the infant and young child should experience a warm, intimate, and continuous relationship to his mother (or mother-substitute) in which both find satisfaction and enjoyment. It is this complex, rich, and rewarding relationship with the mother in the early years, varied in countless ways by relations with the father and with siblings, that underlies the development of character and of mental health.' (1)

These conclusions are now widely accepted by professional workers, both medical and non-medical, in the field of mental health. The recommendations made in this present book are, it is believed, no more than their logical application to one particular problem, namely that of separation from the mother, which is the consequence for most young children of a period in hospital.

During the ten years' work of the Unit, as the member concerned with work in hospitals and sanatoria, I have observed many young children before, during, and after a stay in hospital, including a number with whom research contact has been maintained since they were first observed as long-stay patients in a sanatorium in 1948. Although the Unit is primarily concerned with the scientific study of personality development, and only indirectly with the practical issues of child care, it has been impossible for me to make observations in the hospital setting without becoming concerned with them. The problems set by the behaviour of young patients during and after a stay in hospital have therefore been discussed at length both with hospital staffs and with parents. Hospitals in Europe and America have also been visited to study practice connected with the care of sick children elsewhere; and there has been much correspondence with professional groups in various parts of the world in an exchange of information and opinion on the subject. A number of relevant publications have been issued or are pending (1, 2, 3, 4, 5, 6, 7, 8, 9, 10, 11).

Since the evidence shows that it is with children up to four years of age that the main mental health hazards lie, the explorations of the Unit have been directed mainly to this group, and this book is therefore primarily concerned with children in this age range.

The scope and content of this book, and its length, are substantially those of a memorandum that I wrote on behalf of the Tavistock Clinic and the Tavistock Institute of Human Relations for submission to the committee appointed by the Central Health Services Council (the 'Platt Committee') 'to make a special study of the arrangements made in hospitals for the welfare of children in hospital—as distinct from their medical and nursing treatment—and to make suggestions which could be passed on to hospital authorities'. The Chairman of that committee, Sir Harry Platt, and senior officers at the Ministry of Health, have encouraged the independent publication of the memorandum so that it may achieve the widest possible audience. In making only minor revisions I have resisted the temptation to elaborate or develop any of the themes in many directions that would be possible in a more ambitious publication. I have not, for example, discussed what illness, pain, or surgery, may mean to a child.

JAMES ROBERTSON

ACKNOWLEDGEMENTS

The author is indebted to colleagues in the Child Development
Research Unit of the Tavistock Clinic and Tavistock Institute
of Human Relations, and in particular to Dr John Bowlby, for
discussions during which the ideas set out in the first section
dealing with The Young Child in Hospital were clarified.
Discussions with Barbara Weller, Tutor, St. Mary's Hospital,
London, helped greatly to sort out the problems of nurse
training dealt with in the Postscript. Officers of the General
Nursing Council and the Royal College of Nursing were also
generous of their time, but the views expressed in this book
are not to be attributed to them.

The Unit has received financial support from the National
Health Service (the Central Middlesex, Paddington, and
St. Charles Group Hospital Management Committees; the
North West Regional Hospital Board); the Sir Halley Stewart
Trust; the International Children's Centre; the Josiah Macy, Jr.
Foundation; the Trustees of Elmgrant; the Foundations Fund
for Research in Psychiatry; and the Grant Foundation, Inc.;
and has also worked on contract with the Regional Office for
Europe of the World Health Organization. To all of these
thanks are due. Further opportunities were afforded to the
author for study and observation in the U.S.A. and Canada by
his appointment as a short-term consultant to W.H.O. in 1953,
and by many subsequent visits to the U.S.A. and Continental
Europe.

FOREWORD TO THE FIRST EDITION

JAMES ROBERTSON's *Young Children in Hospital* is an important publication. It is an authoritative review of a problem of great practical concern to everyone interested in the well-being of children. The views expressed derive not only from the author's special experience, but also from that of a group that has been engaged for ten years on research in child development. It clearly presents a most important psychological principle and then in a practical and realistic way makes explicit the implications of this principle for hospital practice.

In one way this publication marks the end of an epoch; in another it shows what we can work for from now on. It is difficult to realize today how different our approach to the care of children in hospital is now as compared with ten years ago. There was then, as now, much kindly feeling; but the underlying ideas determining our management of children's wards have undergone radical changes. This has been due partly to the reassessments that accompanied the upheavals of war, including the evacuation of children from big towns; the 'hospital class' patient is no longer a species apart, for full employment has rubbed out the line between Disraeli's 'two worlds'; and perhaps most important of all, Freud's discoveries have become a part of our general understanding and psychology has become interesting. Today all theories of child growth accept that the early experiences of children are of enormous significance for their later development. Those of us with clinical experience know well that the disturbing things in hospitalization include not only the obviously alarming events, such as anaesthetics and operations, but also separation from the mother, and that this itself is disturbing and sometimes lastingly so.

In many ways the care of young children in hospital has vastly improved in the last ten years; for example, daily visiting is nearly universal. Now we have to ensure that the *quality* of the care given is still further improved; and, for this, a deeper understanding of the problems involved is essential. Herein lies the great value of James Robertson's book and his exposition of the important principle which should determine what we do. Some who read it may feel that the case is overstated, the dangers exaggerated. Nevertheless, as Dr. John Bowlby said in a letter to *Lancet*, on March 1st, 1958 (in which he discusses some of the findings of a systematic follow-up study), although it may be mistaken to say that children who suffer deprivation in early life *commonly* develop lasting emotional disorders, it remains true that *some* suffer grave damage and others lesser damage from separation experience, so that 'the separation of a young child from his mother figure is not to be undertaken without weighty reasons and then only provided there is a suitable and stable substitute available'.

One of James Robertson's previous publications, the film *A Two-Year-Old Goes to Hospital*, was disturbing to many in the hospital professions when it was first shown in 1952. In 1958 there are probably few who do not accept that the film showed a fairly typical example of the distress caused to a young patient by separation from her mother.

This book takes us a stage further. Simultaneously with the publication of the book there will be released James Robertson's new film entitled *Going to Hospital with Mother*, which shows persuasively how practicable as well as desirable it is to admit mothers to hospital with children under four years of age. The book deals also with the occasions on which the mother is not present, as in fever hospitals and long-stay hospitals, and suggests steps we can take for practical preventive mental hygiene in these situations too.

As a children's physician I welcome this book for it is in a tradition of rational and humane care of children in hospital to which some children's physicians in this country, such as James Spence and D. W. Winnicott, contributed largely from its early stages. It is the more welcome for reporting evidence of productive cooperation between psychological workers and workers in children's hospitals. I hope that all of us—doctors, nurses, those concerned with hospital administration, and members of the public—who have responsibility for the care of children in hospital, will read this book. From it we can receive a fresh and a more sustained impetus to our efforts for their lasting welfare. I am very glad this book is being published for if its contents are acted upon we can make a valuable contribution not only to the happiness of children but also to the mental health of this country in the future.

RONALD MAC KEITH, D.M., F.R.C.P.
Physician to Children's Department
Guy's Hospital

'For most children under four years it is our observation that no amount of love and understanding will make up for the absence of the mother. When doctors realize how inextricably emotional welfare is bound up with physical welfare, provisions will be made for a parent to stay with the hospitalized child. If only in the interests of physical well-being, a consideration of the child's emotional needs must eventually take precedence over rules, schedules, and polish on the floor.'

Reducing Emotional Trauma in Hospitalized Children
Departments of Pediatrics and Anesthesiology, Albany Medical College, N.Y.

'Paediatrics is concerned with something more than nursing and the treatment of children. It includes encouraging the mother to develop her own skills by which she remains the chief instrument of child care. The mother is equipped for her duties by developing sensitivities to danger beyond the range of normal feelings. She will hear the whimper of a child in a distant bedroom when other ears are deaf. She will awake instantly to the needs of her child when strangers would do no more than stir slowly in their sleep.'

The Purpose of the Family
Sir James Spence,
Nuffield Professor of Child Health,
University of Durham

The Young Child in Hospital

THE NEED FOR A GUIDING PRINCIPLE

In recent years there has been a marked trend towards 'humanizing' the care of young children in hospital. Amenities are being improved—there is increased visiting, provision of playrooms and teachers, and general brightening of surroundings—but it is clear that these are rarely introduced as part of a coherent approach to meeting the child's emotional needs. If innovations are to be comprehensive and consistent with each other they must derive from a unifying principle and not be assembled on an *ad-hoc* basis.

To illustrate by analogy, in physical medicine there is a principle of asepsis to which all provisions and procedures within a hospital must conform—from the sterilizing of the surgeon's instruments to the cleansing of the kitchen table. Recommendations regarding physical hygiene are not made only with reference to those items that are obviously dirty or that happen to catch the doctor's eye. The principle of asepsis is employed to coordinate all aspects of the *physical* health of the patient.

If a comparable psychological principle of child care were accepted it would be similarly applied to all aspects of the care and management of young patients in the interests of their *mental* health. But since this unifying

1

principle is not yet accepted there is much confusion and disagreement about the nature of the problem and much inconsistency of practice both between and within hospitals. Kind intention is an important factor but of itself no more a sufficient guide than it was in the days before the discovery of the principle of asepsis. Deeper knowledge and understanding is necessary.

There are two overlapping approaches to the subject. There is that of the psychiatrist (and all those who work with him—psychologists, sociologists, and social workers), who is concerned about preventive mental health and knows that a hospital experience has dangers of emotional trauma for the young child; and that of the doctor, nurse, and administrator who, although sometimes in difficulty over evaluating the evidence that important considerations of mental health are involved, recognize that young children are usually unhappy while in hospital and are commonly disturbed in their behaviour for a time at least after their return home. The common ground between the psychological and the traditional approaches is the recognition of current distress and the wish to make children in hospital as happy as possible.

The limitation of the traditional approach is that, being empirical, it takes account only of those matters which attract immediate notice. As is obvious from the current variations in hospital practice, not only do different things come to the notice of different people but even agreed phenomena of behaviour are understood and dealt with in different ways. (One of the most obvious examples of this is that two people seeing that a young child cries at the end of visiting time may make contrary recommendations —the one that the mother should stop visiting, the other that she should continue to visit.)

On the other hand, serious distress may be overlooked

because its expression is inhibited or distorted, because it does not take the manifest form of loud crying, and/or because the staff have become habituated to it and tend to equate distress with tears and contentment with absence of tears. The film *A Two-Year-Old Goes to Hospital* (4, 6, 7, 21) (see p. 20 for summary narrative) shows that a young child can be intensely affected yet have such control over the expression of feeling that the subtler indications of distress could readily be overlooked—and therefore escape the notice and good intention of the empiricist. Optimal methods of caring for young children in hospital can be created only if they are based on an adequate understanding of the nature of the young child and his emotional needs.

THE DEPENDENCY OF THE YOUNG CHILD

The young child in the ordinary family is characterized by total dependency on his parents—particularly on his mother. Although it may appear that in the first few months it does not matter by whom he is handled or by how many people, provided he is fed and made physically comfortable, it would be rash to assume that this is really the case. Studies in progress may well confirm that to be tended by several people in the first months is most disadvantageous (54). However, there is no doubting that before the end of the first year he is very discriminating and almost exclusively attached to his mother—or to the nannie or other woman who mothers him.

In the child of two, for instance, the sense of security and expectations of satisfaction are vested in both parents; but in this phase he is much closer to the mother for obvious reasons related to her biological and social function. He is by no means content to be fed and tended by anyone; he appreciates his mother as a particular person and has a hunger for her love and presence that is as great as his body's hunger for food. She is his whole world, and the little excursions he makes beyond her are rooted in confidence that she is nearby to give him full protection. He has been weaned from the breast, but is still unweaned from complete dependence on the protection and love of this one person. His attachment to her is fiercely possessive, selfish, and intolerant of frustration. And not only has he few ways of expressing his feelings, but he has few ways of understanding what is happening to him. He has little understanding of his environment. To him his parents are omnipotent, can protect him from all harm. He is not far from his mother's skirts all day, and in this close relationship she acts intuitively to meet his physical and emotional needs. In his behaviour he shows his belief not only in his parents' ability to protect him from all harm, but also in their wish to do so—their love and goodwill towards him. They make his world stable and secure.

There is in the young child an urge towards sociability, towards loving and being loved, and it is the proper function of the early environment to allow these to develop and become established in a healthy way. The ordinary family provides this optimal environment in the most natural way. The family is a microcosm of the larger society in which the child will one day be an adult; and if in this critical phase he feels secure and loved, has the experience that love is reciprocated and trust justified, it is likely that in later years he will face life with confidence and with a capacity for good social relationships that are an extension of his early experience.

4

IF HE GOES TO HOSPITAL

If at this critical stage of development, when he has such a possessive and passionate need for his mother and is so blindly trustful of his parents, he is admitted alone to hospital (or indeed to any residential institution), he experiences a serious failure of that environment of love and security hitherto provided by his family, and which we know to be a necessary experience if he is to be a loving, trustful, and secure person in later life.

At this age he is too young to understand that there can be any reason of illness or domestic emergency to justify the loss of his mother's care. Any glimmering of understanding he may have shown before admission is swept away by the tidal wave of his imperative need and he becomes inconsolable and impervious to reassurance. All he knows is that the mother he needs so intensely, the mother who *should* respond to his cries, is not there. He is grief-stricken and angry against those who, to his limited understanding, have let him down.

RECOGNITION OF DISTRESS

The manifest distress of these young patients is now widely recognized and there is a common wish to find means of mitigating it. But for the psychologically trained the matter is more urgent than the softening of an experience for humane reasons. There is evidence that the distress which is shown, and which is increasingly recognized in its more manifest forms, is potentially damaging to the child because among its elements are anger against those he loves and distrust of their attitudes towards him. He has no understanding of the cause of his experience, and can only feel rage and—if able to impute motives—lack of love for him in those he loved and trusted.

When young children return from hospital they are almost invariably anxious and difficult in their behaviour, especially towards their mothers. They sleep badly, go back in their toilet training, panic if mother goes even momentarily out of sight, and have outbursts of aggression against her as if angry with her.

It appears that with tactful handling the disturbances following short separations disappear in a few days or weeks. (The effects of lengthy separations are more serious and will be referred to on p. 14ff.) But there are many children in whom the disturbances persist for much longer, and some who although seemingly recovered can be made anxious by incidents or objects which remind them of the separation situation. The sense of security that should be established in these first years may be shaken by even a short separation from the mother—especially if there also was an operation—as if the immature mental structure could not master the intensity of disturbance and remains in some degree impaired (8, 33) (as an example, see p. 21, Laura).

It is paradoxical that when a young child needs his mother most, when he is ill and perhaps in pain, she is generally not allowed to be with him for more than brief visits—the paradox being that in this situation the staffs of hospitals tend to apply quite different judgements from those they would apply in family life. The sick child at home is seen to need his mother and no one else—but if he comes to hospital his mother is said to 'upset' him. It is also remarkable that although everyone who has lived in a family must be aware of the utter dependence of the young child on his mother, and although it has for many years been common knowledge in the community that young children are acutely unhappy in hospital and are often 'changed' for the worse on return, until recently little attention has been given to the matter in medical and nursing literature—and still all too little in the training of doctors and nurses. Although much evidence has been available in recent years, and the problem is seen to be world-wide, there are many who continue to belittle its significance.

The few systematic studies so far made by hospital units have invariably confirmed that there is an acute problem for the under-fours (19, 23, 27, 29, 32, 44, 50). They are independently agreed that reaction to loss of the parents is the most common manifestation. Several put reaction to anaesthetics and operations next. All but one have follow-up data, where again there is agreement that the great majority of young patients are disturbed and regressed in their behaviour for varying periods after returning home.

Examples

(a) Prugh *et al.* (44), in the most adequate study yet published, report on 100 child patients admitted to an American hospital for mainly medical reasons and with an average stay of 8 days.

The Control Group consisted of 50 children dealt with according to traditional practices of ward management. (Parents could visit once weekly for two hours, and had little encouragement to participate in the ward care of the child. There was no organized programme involving a preventive approach to problems of adjustment.) Of these children, 92 per cent exhibited reactions of a degree indicating significant difficulties in adaptation (moderate and severe categories). Furthermore, on return home 92 per cent of this group showed 'significant disturbances in behaviour not present prior to hospitalization'. Three months later 58 per cent, and six months later 15 per cent of this group remained significantly disturbed in their behaviour.

The Experimental Group consisted of 50 children studied after the management of the ward had been re-organized. (This included daily visiting and participation by the parents in ward care of their child during visits, early ambulation where medically feasible, a special play programme by a nursery schoolteacher, psychological preparation for and support during potentially emotionally traumatic diagnostic and therapeutic procedures, and regular ward management conferences to coordinate the efforts of all professional personnel involved in the care of the sick child.) Of these 50 children, 68 per cent were significantly disturbed in hospital, and on return home the same percentage showed 'significant disturbances in behaviour not present prior to hospitalization' (as opposed to 92 per cent in the Control Group); 44 per cent remained significantly disturbed 3 months later (as opposed to 58 per cent in the Control Group). Proper follow-up of this group was not possible after the 3-month period, but it is the impression of the authors that at 6 months the incidence of significant disturbance was much less than in the Control Group.

Three findings of this study are of special interest for our present purpose:

(i) That although the improvement in ward management greatly reduced the incidence of children significantly disturbed, it still remained high.

(ii) That 'children of 3 years of age and under showed the highest incidence of reaction of severe degree'.

(iii) That the improved conditions of ward management under which the Experimental Group were cared for benefited the older rather than the younger children. *It was principally the younger children who continued to show significant disturbance.*

(*b*) Vaughan (50) reports a comparative study of 40 children admitted to a British hospital for 5 days for an eye operation (strabismus).

The Control Group consisted of 20 children who were dealt with routinely. Of these 40 per cent were 'disturbed' in the ward, 65 per cent showed disturbance a week after discharge, and 55 per cent were still disturbed 6 months later.

The Experimental Group consisted of 20 children matched with their opposite numbers in the Control Group in respect of social background, age, sex, and intelligence. These children were 'prepared' in special interviews with the psychiatrist on the first, third, and fifth days in hospital, with ample opportunity for discussion, explanation, and reassurance. Of these, 55 per cent were 'disturbed' in the ward, 30 per cent showed disturbance a week after discharge, and 15 per cent were still disturbed 6 months later.

But Vaughan reports that although in the Experimental Group 'children of over 4 years had benefited considerably' from the improved handling, '*it is a disquieting observation that all the [four] children under 4 years were still disturbed 6 months after discharge from the ward*'.

Although the studies by Prugh and Vaughan cannot be directly compared because of certain differences in the age structure of the samples and in the criteria used, they have as a common finding that the distress of younger patients was eased little if at all by improved management which significantly reduced the incidence of disturbance in the older children.

To quote from *Reducing Emotional Trauma in Hospitalized Children: A Three-Year Study of* 140 *Tonsillectomized Children* by the Departments of Pediatrics and Anesthesiology at Albany Medical College, Albany, N.Y., (19) with which we believe all the authors referred to on p. 7 will be in agreement:

'For most children under four years it is our observation that no amount of love and understanding will make up for the absence of the mother. When doctors realize how inextricably the emotional welfare is bound up with physical welfare, provisions will be made for a parent to stay with the hospitalized child. If only in the interest of physical well-being, a consideration of the child's emotional needs must eventually take precedence over rules, schedules, and the polish on the floor.'

These are most valuable studies and it is to be hoped that more will follow. But in their broad generalizations they do no more than confirm what is common knowledge in the community—that with negligible exceptions which can be accounted for, every young child parted from his mother by admission to hospital (or, indeed, to any residential institution) reacts by fretting grievously for her. Anyone who cares to raise the topic where ordinary folk meet, in parent-teacher associations and Co-operative Guilds, will soon have an abundance of confirmatory anecdotes.

No criticism is here implied because hospital staffs tend to be slower than ordinary lay people in acknowledging the existence and seriousness of the problem, and certainly no imputation of indifference and inhumanity. But if we look at some of the reasons for the present situation we may understand something more of the problem and the best solutions to it.

First, the initial distress shown by young patients is so commonplace that staff, whatever their initial reaction, feel bound in the end to accept it as inevitable, and to consider later fretting as another inevitable and insignificant phase to be passed through. The tacit assumption is that since every young patient frets at first it is inevitable and cannot be of much consequence.

The second reason is that the distress of the newly admitted young patient is so painful to see that a defensive undervaluation and professional neutrality towards the phenomenon tends to develop—especially if there seems to be no adequate way to deal with it—just as anyone will gradually become less sensitive to a painful situation in everyday life which is recurrent and appears to be unavoidable. It would be intolerable for the nurse or doctor to be as affected by each instance of fretting as by the first, and the tendency to defensive ignoring will continue until more constructive ways of dealing with the distress in young patients are recognized and adopted.

The third reason, and perhaps the most important, is that the young patient can present a picture that is deceptively reassuring. Although he frets bitterly at the beginning of hospitalization he commonly manages in time—perhaps after a few hours, days, or weeks—to appear cheerful or at least placid and amenable. Staff are then tempted to believe that he no longer misses his parents, has 'forgotten' his mother, and is none the worse for his experience. He has then 'settled in'.

11

'SETTLING-IN'

The phenomenon of 'settling-in' is deceptive, and any onlooker might be misled into thinking that a 'settled' young child has accommodated satisfactorily and needs no further thought—though nothing is more certain than that the same quiet and 'settled' child will show by his behaviour on getting home that his contentment in hospital was a façade. (For example, see p. 28, Patricia.) The only valid criterion of a 'settled' or 'happy' young patient would be that when he returned home he picked up where he left off, with little sign that he had been away. There are no studies showing that this ever happens with young children for whom hospitalization means separation from mother.

Since the process of 'settling' gives clues to the danger that hospitalization holds for the young child, it is worth looking more closely at it. On the face of things it seems strange that the young child with a normally intense and exclusive attachment to his mother should 'forget' her, and at least open to question whether it is a good thing that he should do so. My observations have shown three main phases in the process of 'settling'—Protest, Despair, Denial.

Protest. In this initial phase, which may last from a few hours to several days, the young child has a strong conscious need of his mother and the expectation, based on previous experience, that she will respond to his cries. He is grief-stricken to have lost her, is confused and frightened by unfamiliar surroundings, and seeks to recapture her by the full exercise of his limited resources. He has no understanding of his situation, and is distraught with fright and urgent desire to find his mother. He will often cry loudly, shake the cot, throw himself about, and look

12

eagerly towards any sight or sound that might prove to be his missing mother. He may reject the attentions of nurses.

Despair, which gradually succeeds Protest, is characterized by a continuing conscious need of his mother coupled with an increasing hopelessness. He is less active, and may cry monotonously and intermittently. He is withdrawn and apathetic, makes no demands on the environment, and is in a state of deep mourning for his mother—grief of the greatest intensity. This is the quiet stage which is some-times erroneously presumed to mean that distress has lessened, that he is 'settling-in'. It is also the stage which has caused so much controversy about the merits of visiting— 'He was quite settled until his mother came'— an argument which implies that the visiting mother caused the ensuing upset, and overlooks the possibility that the visit merely brought to the surface intense grief and anger that were becoming sealed over. As mentioned above, the same child will show on return home that no matter how amenable he had become in hospital his security and trust in his mother have been disturbed. The three- or four-year-old, being in the upper range of this age group and therefore slightly more mature, may have some understanding that mother comes at the end of each day (if she does), and get a fragment of consolation from it; but even he will react with anxiety and resentment on return home. The still younger child, bound to the mother and lacking all time-sense and understanding, cannot cope with the eternities between visits—and even daily visiting touches only the fringe of his need.

Some children who are in hospital for a short time only will reach the stage of Despair though others will go home in the stage of Protest. But if the young child stays longer

13

in typical conditions in which he is cared for by a variety of nurses, he will enter the phase of:

Denial. In this phase, which gradually succeeds Despair, he shows more interest in his surroundings and this may be welcomed as a sign that he is becoming 'happy'. It is, however, a danger signal. Because the child cannot tolerate the intensity of distress he begins to make the best of his situation by repressing his feelings for his mother. He deals drastically with his feeling for the mother who has failed to meet his needs, particularly his need of her as a person to love and be loved by. Then he is free to take such satisfactions, food, and attention as the ward can offer. It may then be thought that because he smiles and responds to play he has 'settled' in the sense that all is well. But it will often be seen that when his mother comes he seems hardly to know her, and no longer cries when she leaves—on the face of it a peaceful situation, but on reflection surely a disconcerting thing that a child so young should seem to have lost his love for and attachment to his mother.

It is disquieting that these processes of denial can occur in long-stay children even if they see their mothers daily.

Another aspect of this common phenomenon is shown by the child who on the day of discharge will not leave Sister's arms to go to his mother. This is sometimes taken to mean that he enjoyed the ward so much that he is reluctant to go home; but who can really believe that a young child could prefer such a situation to being with his mother unless something had gone wrong inside him? Observations of his behaviour after return home confirm this. Usually he thaws out gradually and then shows typical clinging and fearful behaviour. And if taken back to the ward for a visit he clings tightly to mother and shuns Sister and everything which reminds him of his stay in hospital.

Finally, if his stay is lengthy, and if the nursing system is of the usual kind, he will in time seem not only not to need his mother but not to need any mothering at all—a peculiar and remarkable state which if it were seen in a child in the family would rightly cause considerable concern. Yet it can be seen at any time in many long-stay children's wards, where it draws little or no comment.

As was said earlier, the young child has a primary need of a close and loving relationship to his mother or to one other taking her place. Recognition of this primary need is intuitive with the ordinary person. If a child were to lose his mother by her death or illness, those around him would know that his grievous need was best met by attaching him to one person who would substitute for the mother he had lost. They would not think to give him into the custody of a rota of neighbours, passing him from one to the other through the ensuing weeks and months. Without reference to theory they would know intuitively that the right thing to do for a motherless child is to attach him to *one* substitute mother.

But if he loses his mother's care by going into hospital, this deep-rooted intuitive knowledge of his needs is usually unapplied in what happens there. Instead of being given into the care of one nurse—or a minimum number of nurses—he meets the very fate that he would have been spared had he been orphaned. He has a rota of custodians instead of one. In the first twenty-four hours he will be handled by a succession of nurses who will variously bathe, feed, and change him. Even if Sister eases his first days by having him 'specialled' by one nurse, the traditional system of staff organization will in time take over. The nurses will be on shift duty, and within a very few weeks most of them will have moved on to other wards in the course of training and other nurses will have taken their place. And among this bewildering variety of nurses, no matter how kindly each one may be in her fragment of care, there will be no one whose job it is to cherish the child and give him that experience of a continuing relationship of love and security which is necessary to him in that stage of development (30).

Most hospital wards are thus quite impersonal in the young child's experience of them, no matter how devoted and hardworking the staff. If the child's care is divided among many people, his need of attachment is *ipso facto* not met. If he has no opportunity to find a human being who will substitute for his mother (the ward sister has too many charges to meet this need at all adequately), or if he has the experience of becoming attached to a series of nurses each of whom leaves and so repeats for him the pain and sense of rejection of the original loss of his mother, he will in time act as if neither mothering nor contact with humans has much significance for him. He will learn by bitter experience that it is folly to become attached to any nurse, because nurses move on to other wards; thus, after a series of upsets at losing several nurses to whom in turn he has given his trust and warm affection, he will gradually commit himself less and less to succeeding nurses and in time will stop altogether taking the risk of investing love and dependence in anyone. He will no longer be upset when nurses change or leave, because no one nurse matters to him. He will cease to show feeling when his parents come and go on visiting days; and he may cause them pain when they realize that although he has little interest in them as particular people

16

he has an avid interest in the presents they bring. Nevertheless, most deceptively, he will appear cheerful and apparently easy and unafraid of anyone.

In this final stage of adaptation, which may be reached in some months or a year or so after the separation which initially caused him so much distress, he will seem to the casual eye to be thoroughly adjusted to his situation. This is the little three- or four-year-old who charms visiting doctors and administrators because he is so bright and sociable and easy in his relationships. But if the visitor were to sit in the ward for a day he would see that this sociability is superficial and promiscuous, that the child is attached to no one—a state that is highly abnormal for the young child and that, if it becomes established as a feature of his personality, will make him a serious misfit in later life.

It cannot be too strongly emphasized that the picture which such children make, although superficially sociable and contributing to the general brightness of the long-stay ward, is quite unlike that of children who grow up in the family. These hospitalized children allow human beings to come and go without regret; and, instead of being secure and attached to their parents and as full of demands and jealousies as the normal young child, do not seem to care much whether they have parents or not. They have little satisfaction in relationships and enjoy people only in so far as they offer diversion and the satisfaction of an excessive interest in material things on to which their frustrated need for love becomes displaced. But since the manifest behaviour of these children is not troublesome and they are members of a 'happy' community, they draw little comment from staff except in respect of their illnesses. They are easier to manage than in the earlier stages of their separation. But from the

aspect of mental health their situation is most unsatisfactory. Through prolonged lack of stable affectionate
relationships of the kind children normally experience in
the family, their capacity for loving attachment has
become impaired. This, coupled with an excessive interest
in material satisfactions, can persist as an undesirable
character trait (8, 9).

Although a follow-up study done by our Unit (3) has
shown that fewer young children than was at one time
believed develop psychopathic or affectionless characters
through severe deprivation caused by long periods in
hospital, it did nothing to cast doubt on the many studies
which indicate that *some* children in their personality
development suffer grave damage and others lesser
damage from a separation experience. Furthermore,
since there are no ready and reliable methods of estimating
the degree of residual disturbance there is no cause for
complacency (2).

But whether the likelihood of permanent impairment is
great or small, what is certain is that the aftermath of a
lengthy stay in hospital in the early years is commonly
an extended period of serious maladaptation and unhappiness for the child, and serious difficulties for the
family to whose care he is returned. Even if in the course
of years the child is one of those whose mental recovery
is complete, the cost in terms of stress, family friction,
and wasted months or years is high.

I have a small series of first-hand longitudinal studies
of children observed during and after lengthy periods
in hospital begun before the age of four. The hospital
was well run by contemporary standards and the staff
conscientious and kindly, but it was nevertheless an
environment which did not meet the young child's primary

need of a warm and continuous relationship to a mother figure. The behaviour of all of these children made great difficulties for their families for some years afterwards. Eight years after discharge the individual outcomes are varied, but each child has a residue of impairment of personality and mental functioning of a kind that was broadly predictable on the basis of their emotional states at time of discharge from the long-stay hospital. Among the features to be found in varying degree and combination are—difficulty in making and sustaining relationships; shallowness of attachment; immaturity; excessive stubbornness and self-centredness; distractibility and inability to concentrate, resulting in inadequate use of intellectual endowment. (These children will be presented at length in a forthcoming publication. For a summarized example see p. 32, Barbara.)

TWO MAIN DANGERS OF HOSPITALIZATION

There is a considerable literature on the meaning of illness, pain, and surgery to young children, but although these are a potential source of psychological disturbance their consideration is not within the scope of this book. We are here dealing mainly with the thesis that the young child has a primary need of 'a warm, intimate, and continuous relationship to his mother (or permanent mother-substitute) in which both find satisfaction and enjoyment'; and with the corollary that it is therefore a serious matter to separate the young child from his mother.

To summarize the first part of this book, a stay in hospital without maintaining adequate contact with his mother exposes the young child to two main dangers:

The Traumatic, in which the shock of losing the mother, especially if this is associated with painful investigations and operations, may be more than the immature mental structure of the young child can tolerate—and may therefore so affect it that he is left with feelings of insecurity and hostility against the environment. These may stay with him for a long time, in some instances probably permanently (17, 19, 32, 35, 44).

Experiences of pain and fright which might overwhelm and scar the young mind may be so mitigated by the presence of the mother as to be made harmless (10, 11, 26). Nevertheless, whether or nor the mother stays with the child, it is essential to rationalize procedures of handling the child to achieve a minimum of disturbance.

To the Traumatic the passage of time can add:

The Deprivational, in which lengthy separation from the mother undergone in a traditionally organized hospital ward may result in prolonged deprivation of maternal-type care (i.e. care by one mother figure) and a consequent and serious impoverishment of the personality (1, 2, 3, 9, 33, 34). It is essential to find ways of preventing such gross deficiency in the experience of long-stay patients.

THREE CHILDREN
NOTES FROM A CASEBOOK

In this section is presented material from my observations to illustrate some of the points in the foregoing.

(a) A SHORT STAY IN HOSPITAL

Most children of under four, particularly those between eighteen months and three years, react initially with acute fretting when admission to hospital entails separation from the mother. Then, in the course of hours or days, they become 'settled'. However, at the beginning and end of visiting times they tend to cry—which suggests that their 'settledness' is a cover for continuing distress which is no longer overtly expressed. Not uncommonly the passage of time also results in gradual lessening of active interest in the parents—as if the child, unable to understand his situation, begins to lose faith in the love and good intention of the parents who do not take him home. On return home after even only a few days in hospital there is usually a period of days, weeks, or longer during which the child shows by clinging, temper tantrums, aggression against the mother, and by other forms of insecure behaviour, the effects of the interrupted relationship with his mother.

The first child, Laura, selected at random for a scientific film record of separation behaviour, was highly intelligent and had an unusual degree of control over the expression of feeling. When admitted to hospital she did not react with the initial abandoned fretting that is typical of the age group (and which is illustrated on p. 32 in 'Barbara') but there is no doubting the stress she was under. Laura's behaviour is described in the form of a summary of the film, *A Two-Year-Old Goes to Hospital*.

LAURA: In hospital for eight days for hernia repair at age 2 years 5 months.

Laura is 2 years 5 months old, a first child and so far an only one, though a second baby is due in four months' time. She is intelligent, mature, and for her age has unusual control over the expression of feeling. She rarely cries. She has never been out of her mother's care, but in two days' time she will go into hospital for eight days to have an umbilical hernia repaired.

First Day in Hospital. Laura's parents have tried to prepare her for going into hospital, but she is too young to understand that she will leave the care of her mother. Therefore when she meets the admitting nurse in the hospital ward she is friendly and cheerful and unafraid. But when the nurse takes her away and undresses her to be given a bath she screams for her mummy. But her mother is far away in the waiting-room and does not come. In ten minutes Laura's exceptional control over the expression of feeling asserts itself and she is apparently calm.

She is put into a cot and again cries bitterly when the nurse takes her temperature—'Don't like it. I want my mummy.' A few minutes later mother comes to say good-bye. Laura begins sobbing, then her face becomes set and solemn and apprehensive. She cannot understand what is happening, but makes no protest. Mother leaves for her consolation a piece of blanket she has had since infancy and which she calls her 'baby'. (Like many young children Laura gets comfort from a favourite 'cuddly toy' and usually goes to sleep holding and sometimes sucking it.) Throughout her stay in hospital this 'blanket baby' and her teddy bear make a link with home and are clung to when she is sad or frightened.

When alone in the hospital cot she appears calm, and to the casual eye would seem 'settled'; but if a kindly person stops to talk with her her feelings break through. The camera shows that what may easily be taken for calmness is often a façade which cracks to release bitter tears when a friendly nurse makes contact. Occasionally during the day she asks for her mummy, but quietly and without insistence.

When the surgeon comes to have a look at the hernia she is apprehensive and resistive despite his kind manner; she clutches her teddy bear and 'blanket baby' for comfort. And as her hair is brushed at bedtime she asks quietly, once only, 'Where *is* my mummy?' Much later she is still awake and restless, tossing about in her cot and gnawing at teddy bear. She is given a sedative to put her to sleep.

On the Second Day she woke very early and spent most of the morning quietly grizzling in her cot. Occasionally she called out in a plaintive voice to busy nurses as they passed her cot, 'Where has my mummy gone?'

When the camera lights on her during the forenoon she is quiet, but her expression is strained and sad and very different from that of the friendly and cheerful little girl who had been admitted twenty-four hours earlier. Nothing has been done to her yet, but she is showing the stress of being out of her mother's care. She has difficulty in responding to the nurse who comes to play with her, pushes away the toy that is offered, and swallows hard as if controlling herself. Her eyes have narrowed, and her mouth droops. Then the friendly contact with the nurse again causes her feelings to break through and she cries for a short time for her mummy. (Though she cries little throughout her stay in hospital, all the time keeping the expression of her own feelings firmly in check, she takes great interest in other children who cry—as if they cry for her who is too controlled to cry.) Shortly afterwards a rectal anaesthetic is administered. The nurses are kindly, but the strange experience in a strange place frightens Laura. She is then taken to the operating theatre.

Thirty minutes after she has come round from the anaesthetic her parents visit. Laura is very distressed—'I want to go home'—and tries to get to her mother; but a nurse restrains her because of the stitches. She turns away from her parents in despair and covers her eyes. Being too young to have any understanding she is acutely disappointed that her mother does not take her into her arms. Her parents, frustrated in their impulse to touch and comfort Laura, feel helpless. Unable to console her, they try to jolly her. But this has no meaning for the child. As they leave she looks subdued and perplexed, as if overcome by the (to her) inexplicable fact that the parents who have hitherto protected her are leaving her alone in her distress.

Third Day. In the morning she is seen quietly clutching her teddy and 'blanket baby', not crying or demanding attention but looking to and fro as if in hope that a familiar person will appear in the strange and busy place. When a nurse comes to play with her she is at first withdrawn; then the contact with a friendly person again causes her suppressed feelings to break through and she cries bitterly for her mummy. When the nurse leaves, her unusual control reasserts itself. But when the nurse returns shortly afterwards we see the same cycle of withdrawal, breakdown into bitter crying, and gradual recovery of composure after the nurse has left. The camera shows her frown and bite a trembling lip in the effort not to cry, and her hands flutter before her eyes. Twenty minutes later her face is still, and she sits quietly looking out at the ward. A 'settled' child. The only movement is in the play of her fingers as they lie in her lap.

In the afternoon her mother visits, but although Laura has wanted her so much she makes no attempt to get to her. Her natural spontaneity towards her mother has been frozen. She seems to have doubts about her mother's goodwill towards her. It is only after fifteen minutes that she thaws out. She becomes increasingly animated and friendly, and is transfigured by a radiant smile seen for the first time in three days. But she does not realize that the mother she has just regained is going to leave her again. When her mother leaves, Laura turns her head away. She does not understand the medical necessity, and for her this is an experience of rejection by her mother. She resists tears, but her distress is shown by the change in her expression and the restless movement of her hands. Although it is the middle of the day she asks to be tucked down with all her treasured possessions from home around her—the 'blanket baby', the teddy bear, the little gifts that her mother had brought. She forbids the nurse to remove the chair on which her mother had been sitting— 'Don't take away my mummy's chair.'

Fifth Day. As the days go by she is increasingly withdrawn and inactive. When her mother visits Laura turns her head away and wipes off her mother's kiss, and although in time she relents she is less animated than on the previous visit. When her mother leaves she cries piteously for a moment, then sits quietly with pursed lips.

On the Sixth Day a boy of three-and-a-half is brought in. Less controlled than Laura, and therefore more typical of the age group, he cries bitterly all afternoon. This disturbs Laura. Her own tears held precariously in check, she keeps looking across at him with a solemn, anxious face. Then she says urgently, 'Why is that boy crying? Go fetch his mummy.' She does not see her own mother that day.

Seventh Day. In the morning, after her stitches have been taken out, she cries in the sister's arms and says plain-

25

tively, 'I want to go home now my tummy's better.' She has remembered the assurance given by her mother four days ago. But when her mother comes that afternoon Laura shows no excitement whatever. Although she is up she makes no attempt to get to her mother, but is subdued and unresponsive. When her father arrives ten minutes later he gets a warmer welcome—she is not angry with him, but only with mother. But on this visit she does not come alive, but remains subdued throughout. Nothing is said to her about going home, and although she knows she should go home now her tummy is better she does not mention it—or once only. As her father prepares to leave she says quietly, and without insistence, 'I come with you,' then seems to ignore his departure. When mother leaves twenty minutes later Laura does not look at her, and does not respond to the cheerful waving, but stands with head bent. She seems thoroughly confused by the failure of her parents to take her home, and at such a tender age she cannot understand it except in terms of their rejection of her.

On the Eighth Day, when mother approaches her cot saying, 'I've come to take you home,' Laura does not react immediately. She watches cautiously and unsmilingly as if unwilling to make the commitment of trusting her mother's words after these many disappointments. Only when her outdoor shoes are produced does she seem convinced of her mother's reliability. She comes to life, dresses eagerly, and insists on collecting every one of her personal possessions to take home.

Epilogue. Like most young children who return from hospital, Laura went through a period of marked anxiety and irritability. She wetted and soiled herself, and was very upset if her mother went even momentarily out of sight—as if fearing she might be abandoned once more. She slept badly, and for the first few nights mother had to sleep in the same bedroom. Laura called out several times in her sleep, 'Don't do it to me. I'm not a naughty girl.' (Sometimes little children misconstrue being in hospital as a punishment for being naughty.)

Although she clung to her mother she was also aggressive towards her—would suddenly punch and scratch as if blaming her for what had happened. Towards father she was consistently friendly, as she was seen to be in the film when he visited her in hospital. At this age he was of much less importance to her than mother. Mother, the one who had been closest to her and who had protected and cared for her in everyday life while father was at work, was therefore the one who got the brunt of her disappointment and anger over being left in hospital.

These disturbances gradually diminished; but six months later, when she got a reminder of hospital, she burst into violent tears and said angrily to her mother, 'Where was you all that time?' Then she turned away from her and cried on her father's shoulder.

Mother said, truly and with dismayed surprise, 'She seems to blame me for something' (4, 6, 7, 21).

(b) A 'SETTLED' CHILD

It is sometimes difficult for the onlooker to believe that a young child who has reached the phase of being 'settled' (that is, being friendly towards the nurses and no longer crying at visiting times) may show considerable disturbance in her behaviour after return home.

Young Children in Hospital

PATRICIA: In hospital for five weeks because of abscess on appendix at age 3 years 9 months. Visited daily.

Project

The ward sister and two doctors attached to the children's ward of a teaching hospital were of the opinion that if a young child showed difficult behaviour on return from hospital it was probably caused by factors unrelated to the experience of being in hospital—mainly that parents were so glad to have their children home that they 'spoiled' them and thus provoked demanding behaviour in their children. Sister and doctors thought that if there had been nothing particularly distressing in the nature of a child's illness or its treatment, and if the child had seemed to make a happy adjustment to the ward and to visiting parents who were sensible people, the prognosis was that this settled attitude would continue without relapse when the child returned home.

They instanced Patricia as a child who had adjusted very well to the ward following a few days of crying when her parents left at the end of visiting time; who then adjusted to her parents' visits and, although always pleased to see them, no longer protested when they left; and whose parents were sensible people who would not provoke bad behaviour by 'spoiling' her when she returned home. Their prognosis was that Patricia's seemingly contented behaviour and good relationship to her parents would continue without special disturbance on her return home. Patricia had been a special favourite in the ward but it was agreed that she had not been indulged to her detriment.

I undertook to visit the home—

    (a) to test this prognosis, and

    (b) to assess, if possible, the extent to which regular daily visiting and a ward which provides teaching and an atmosphere of friendly individual interest in the children (not to the extent of case-assignment nursing), prevented this child of 3 years 9 months from feeling deprived.

Follow-up

Twenty-four days after Patricia's discharge from hospital I visited the home by arrangement, and saw mother, maternal grandmother, and Patricia. We talked for an hour, and the following emerged:

Before Hospital—Patricia had not previously been away from her mother. She was 'A mummy's girl', rather 'clingy' and shy of strangers.

During Hospital—Patricia was visited each evening by one or other parent, and sometimes by maternal grandmother. After the first four occasions she was pleased to see them and did not cry when they left. Mother remarked on how happy Patricia had been in the ward, and how familiar with and attached to the staff.

After Hospital—My informants were very vague at first about what had happened, in part I judged because they were very appreciative of the care and kindness of the ward and did not wish to seem ungrateful, and partly because they did not wish to make critical comments on their child. At first mother went no further than that 'Patricia was a bit defiant for a day or two, then it passed over'; but some time later, after maternal grandmother had said, 'For one week she nearly drove us mad, and I had to lock myself in my room to get away from her,' more details emerged which make it possible to present a clearer but still very incomplete picture of the child's behaviour.

(a) During the first week home she lost much of her independence and insisted on being spoon fed by her mother. She wanted to be 'babied' (she did not regress in cleanliness).

(b) For the whole of the second week her behaviour was very difficult. 'She was into everything.' She seemed deliberately to try out the patience of mother and maternal grandmother (and got the punishment she asked for), and she was always on the verge of tears—ready to cry on the slightest provocation.

(c) Somewhere around the third week her behaviour modified, to the elders' relief because 'she had always been a good easy child'.

(d) She talked a lot about hospital from the time she came home.

Return Visit to the Ward

Four weeks after discharge Patricia returned to Out-Patients for examination, and was then taken to the ward by her mother. She seemed pleased to see children she knew, and to meet the staff again. She was specially glad to see Sister and the doctor who had dealt with her; but she kept a firm grip on her mother's hand and would not go anywhere without her.

That night she woke up crying, saying she was too hot and wanted to get into mother's bed; and next day she was unusually disobedient. A few days later the family went to a pantomime and Patricia would not stay in her seat while mother went for ices. She said, 'I don't want them to take me away again.'

Opinion

Although the behaviour of this child gave no indication of it while she was in hospital, it is clear from the 'baby' spell in the week after discharge that her seemingly perfect adjustment concealed some degree of deprivation which did not become manifest until her mother was again restored to her. It nevertheless also seems likely that daily visiting and the degree of security given by a free and friendly ward somewhat diminished the disturbance of being away from mother—evidenced by Patricia's ability to return to the ward and to show pleasure in renewing acquaintances, although taking the very understandable precaution of keeping a grip on her mother. It is probable that had this child been in a non-visiting ward of different climate from this one she would have shown greater anxiety if brought for a return visit.

(c) A LONG STAY IN HOSPITAL

If a young child is long enough in hospital he will pass through the stages of Protest, Despair, and Denial described on pp. 12-18. To the shock of losing his mother will eventually be added the condition of emotional impoverishment inevitably resulting from a lengthy stay in an environment which does not meet the young child's primary need of a warm, intimate, and continuous relationship with one mother-figure.

The child may then seem well-adjusted to the constantly changing society of the ward; but it is an adjustment significantly lacking in deep attachment to anyone—to transient staff or to visiting parents. On return home in this final stage of emotional impoverishment he will have considerable difficulty in fitting into normal family and social relationships. This maladaptation will usually

31

continue over an extended period, and in some instances at least may leave a permanent residue of impaired capacity for making and sustaining satisfactory relationships. Mental functioning may also be impaired.

BARBARA: In hospital for eighteen months for pulmonary tuberculosis from age 2 years to 3 years 6 months. Visited weekly.

Barbara was brought to the hospital by her parents. She was an attractive little girl with pert face and blonde hair done up in ribbon. It was summer, and she was freshly dressed in a yellow spotted frock with pants to match. While her parents made final arrangements with the ward sister, Barbara ran about the office taking a lively interest in its contents—quite unsuspecting of what was about to happen to her. A nurse removed her, kindly but firmly to an adjoining cubicle, slipped off her pretty dress and stood her in a cot where she was left alone.

Protest. Barbara began a loud screaming. She could catch occasional glimpses of her parents through a small window, and made desperate efforts to attract their attention. The parents were themselves in distress, because they could not respond to Barbara's cries for help. When I left an hour later Barbara was still bellowing at the top of her voice. Her face was livid and tear-stained, and hardly recognizable as that of the fresh-complexioned little girl who an hour previously had been playing happily about, secure in the presence of her mother. The sister picked her up and tried to quieten her, but to no avail. Some 'up' children gathered around, then at a word scattered to their cubicles to bring gifts to divert the new patient. But Barbara was not interested, and continued to scream, watched from the doorway by a group of quite silent children through whose minds may well have flickered recollections of an initial experience of similar kind. Barbara's secure world had suddenly crumbled in the loss of her mother, and at that age the kindness of strangers was no solace to her fear and longing.

That night she slept badly, waking and calling for her mother. When she awoke in the morning she immediately resumed her loud, protesting crying. She refused food, took notice of no one, and could not be consoled. Later that day, the second of her separation, the vigour of her crying had abated; but it still went on. She lay in her cot, sometimes still, sometimes throwing herself about like a person demented. She seemed quite out of her mind in a mixture of protest and despair, and quite withdrawn from her environment.

Despair. Two days later, the fourth of her separation, she was much quieter but still agitated, chewing her fist and incessantly peering about the cubicle, obviously looking for her mother. When anyone opened the cubicle door she paused to look eagerly in that direction, but quickly returned to misery and disregard of her surroundings.

When her parents were allowed to visit on the fifth day she turned away from them and sobbed bitterly into her pillow. She was so desperately miserable, and so bewildered and angry to have been treated thus by the people in whom her love and trust had been vested, that she rejected them as it seemed they had rejected her. The mother and father spent the whole visiting hour coaxing her to take notice of them, and had just succeeded in re-establishing some relationship when the bell went and they had to desert her again. Barbara became frantic. She climbed on to the cot rails and clung so firmly to her father that she had to be removed by force. As her parents hurried from the ward they could hear her piercing screams behind them.

The parents were allowed to visit weekly, and for a month or so the occasions were most painful. During the week Barbara had become placid and amenable, and gave no trouble. But when her parents visited, feelings which might otherwise have been unsuspected came to the surface. Sometimes she buried her face in the pillow and would have nothing to do with them for minutes on end; sometimes she lay and screamed; sometimes she was desperate to get into her mother's arms, but that was not allowed.

Denial. As the weeks passed her behaviour gradually changed in a way which is typical of young children who remain for lengthy periods in such kindly but impersonal surroundings. She began to show less and less distress when her parents paid their weekly visit. She cried and was resentful for a few minutes after their arrival, then quickly brightened and seemed to enjoy their company, and when they left cried again and was restless until a good tea restored her composure. In a later stage she showed neither tears nor resentment when they came, was cheerful throughout the visit, cried briefly when they left but quickly took up some activity as if recovered. Still later she would greet them cheerfully, be active and gay throughout the visit, and wave them a bright good-bye as if she no longer had any wish to be with them; sometimes she would even dismiss them in anticipation of the end of the hour, so that she could get back to play. During the week her behaviour in the ward was increasingly bright and cheerful, and she stopped crying or—as far as anyone noticed—mentioning her parents. But although superficially amiable she was attached to no one. Nurses came

34

and left, but Barbara showed no upset at the many changes. She had in fact withdrawn feeling from the possibility of hurt. She no longer showed disturbances on her parents' weekly visits. When she saw them arrive her face lit up, not, apparently, for their own sakes but because of the diversion they brought, in much the same way as she might greet me if I had a sweet in my pocket. She dug into her mother's bag and enjoyed the toys and sweets she found there; but she showed no warmer interest in her parents than in the transient nurse. She had long ceased to try to be taken in her mother's arms; and even when that was permitted as her health improved she showed no wish for such intimacy. Her mother would sit by her cot and say such things as 'Isn't it a nice mummy who brings you these things, Barbara?'; but Barbara, although superficially bright and easy, did not respond to her mother's wish for a sign of attachment.

Barbara returned home after eighteen months. She proved exceedingly difficult to deal with. A year later she was still hyperactive—ran everywhere, skipped incessantly, could not sit at table—as if full of dammed-up energy that had to be discharged. She was very wilful, did not take account of rebuke, and if frustrated in the slightest would throw temper tantrums of extreme severity—in the home or in the street. She was destructive—would break dishes and damage the walls of the home wantonly and aggressively. She seemed to have no need of affection, shrugged off the attempted caresses of her parents, and would wander away from home. Her appetite for sweets and other tangible satisfaction—as opposed to satisfaction through affectionate relationships—was excessive.

Lest this should appear an extreme picture I should add that it is in fact not at all unusual.

Some Implications for Hospital Practice

PLAINLY, the more that children can be kept out of hospital or nursed at home the better (36). The next best thing is to have mother and child together in hospital. If this can be achieved, the mental health problem of the welfare of young children in hospital is virtually solved. Since the admission of mothers with their children is the optimum provision, we shall begin our considerations there and only then consider how far and in what way other provisions can compensate for the absence of the mother.

ADMISSION OF MOTHER AND CHILD

In less developed countries than ours it is common practice for members of the family to accompany the patient into hospital and there to attend to his comfort while doctors and nurses deal with his illness. (Native doctors and nurses from those areas coming to Britain to attend courses are sometimes at a loss to understand the debate here about what is to them common practice and common sense.) This is only partly a reflection of the simpler organization of hospitals in these parts. More importantly it shows that given the opportunity the human family will act on the intuition that it is good for the morale of the sick person to be looked after by his own kin. It has been observed in parts of eastern Europe that the setting up of modern hospitals with regulations designed to restrict contact between parents and their sick children has been difficult because of the opposition of peasant families to being excluded.

Similar family attitudes are to be found at the other extreme. In Western cultures the sick of the wealthiest and most sophisticated groups are usually cared for in nursing homes and the private wings of hospitals to which their kin have unrestricted access. In particular it is usual for the young children of this privileged group to be accompanied into hospital by mother or by nannie.

Universally, therefore, at the extremes of simplicity and sophistication, those families which are permitted or can obtain the facility show their belief that the sick child should not be parted from his mother. Yet the hospital systems that have developed to serve the greater proportion of the populations of all industrialized countries have severely restricted the contact between the sick child and his mother. The reasons for this are complex and beyond the scope of this short book. It is sufficient to note that the recommendation that ways should be found to keep child and mother together in hospital is not a new one.

Thirty years ago Spence (46, 47, 48) demonstrated the practicability of this method at Newcastle, but his example had few imitators until very recent times. Five years ago the only one known to us was the professor of paediatrics at a hospital in the Balkans who shortly after a visit to Spence at Newcastle set up an experimental unit in which 24 mothers were resident with their babies and young children (39). Careful inquiry at that time discovered no other hospital in Europe or America in which the routine admission of mother and child was advocated and practised, though elsewhere, as in Britain, the facility could be bought. In the Antipodes, 'nursing by the mother' as a positive therapeutic device in the care of babies undergoing operation for cleft palate was initiated by the Pickerills at about the same time as Spence began his work, and has continued with much success (42).

There is no doubt that resistance to the idea has been, and continues to be, great. Three main objections are made:

(*a*) That it is not possible to accommodate mothers until specially designed wards have been built.

(*b*) That mothers would obstruct the work of the ward by their presence and by anxious and unreliable behaviour.

(*c*) That the young patient is more difficult to manage in the presence of his mother, particularly during examination or treatment.

(*a*) It has by now been convincingly demonstrated that there are many wards of traditional design in which mothers and children could be accommodated together, *provided staff decide to do it* and are prepared to modify routine to suit that kind of arrangement. At the Babies Hospital, New-castle, the practice established by Spence is successfully continued with mainly working-class mothers as is the work begun by the Pickerills in New Zealand. More recently several schemes have been reported (10, 16, 25, 26, 37). At Amersham General Hospital, which is well known to me, a ward of traditional design has been adapted to accommodate mothers and young children by the simple expedient of adding a bed and easy chair to the cot and locker which are the usual equipment of cubicles. As is typical of many children's wards, these cubicles line one side of the corridor leading to the open ward and are customarily used to protect babies from cross-infection. At Amersham most are now used for the accommodation of young children and their mothers (10, 37). And in an

American hospital also known to me, in which children sleep four or six to a room, collapsible beds which stow away in day-time are in use for mothers (25, 26). In both instances the improvisations give only minimum facilities to the mothers, but there is no doubt that the great majority of them are contented and grateful for the possibility of staying with their children.

(*b*) The objection that resident mothers would obstruct the work of the ward by their presence, and by anxious and unreliable behaviour, is more difficult to deal with since it is true that all hospital staffs have experience of visiting mothers who are 'awkward'. Instances are given of mothers who complain about trivial things, who cry over their children and make them agitated, who even give sweets and pastries to children on diets. Undoubtedly mothers are sometimes complaining and unreliable at visiting times, but the view which hospital staffs tend to get of mothers is one which is often distorted by the special circumstances in which they are generally seen.

The ordinary mother is usually a competent housewife and if her child is ill at home she will deal with him sensibly under the direction of the family doctor, even when the illness is serious. But like anyone else if she finds herself in a situation that is specially restrictive it is likely she will feel frustrated and show it in behaviour that is unusual for her. This can sometimes be seen in wards which allow visiting once a week only. Mothers will arrive laden with expensive gifts, and during their short hour may make sharp complaints about toys broken or gifts of the previous week that are no longer to be seen. They may even surreptitiously feed harmful titbits to children on special diets although clearly cautioned not to do so.

The reason is not that all of these mothers are irresponsible and ungrateful for the care that is being given, but simply that the strong maternal impulse to show love to their children is so highly frustrated by the restrictions on visiting and on physical contact with their children that they are driven to make the only gestures of love left open to them—to bring extravagant gifts and even to pass forbidden sweets in defiance of their own common sense. The truth of this interpretation of uncharacteristic behaviour by mothers who are ordinarily reasonable beings is found in the experience of those wards which have introduced more frequent visiting. It is then seen that the more contact the mother has with her young child, especially if she is also allowed to do simple things like feeding and washing, the more normal does her behaviour become. The less she is frustrated in the expression of her normal maternal impulses the less is she impelled to bring costly presents to substitute for it or to pop a sweet in her child's mouth to compensate him for her felt shortcomings.

This simple truth of human behaviour, that people behave better when they can express their natural creative impulses than when they are frustrated, explains why mothers in mother-child units are so much more reasonable than is expected by those who have met them only in circumstances of restricted visiting or in out-patient departments. It is not suggested that mothers in mother-child units will always be easy to deal with. They will have times of anxiety, but it will be more appropriate anxiety than develops when they are shut off from participation in the care of their children; and staff who believe in their presence will not find it difficult to give them whatever support and reassurance they need.

There are some wards in which certain selected mothers of under-fours are admitted. The 'anxious' mother is excluded. It is in fact rarely justified to discriminate in this way. The presence of even an 'anxious' mother is infinitely better for the young child than that she should be absent. A mother would need to be very unbalanced indeed before it could reasonably be considered that her presence was to the detriment of her young child. It is a mark of excellence at Amersham that the staff do not presume to discriminate 'good' and 'bad' mothers in this way. The mother of every patient of under-four is invited to come into hospital with him. The conviction that the presence of the ordinary mother, however 'anxious', is good for her child is thus wholeheartedly implemented—and because of this conviction the staff are ready to cope with the range of personalities and temperaments the mothers reveal.

Much of the skill in running a good mothers-in unit will in fact reside in assessing for each mother admitted how far she can be left to carry on in her own way, how far she needs guidance, and to what extent she needs support and reassurance. In principle, the more the ordinary mother can be allowed to be herself the better. She is, after all, the mother who reared the child and who will be looking after him when he leaves hospital, and in matters of ordinary care and the nuances of comfort she knows best what her child needs. It is a good professional rule to let a mother work at her own level, supporting her in her skills and understanding and bolstering her confidence in herself, quietly supplementing her efforts instead of giving detailed directions and cautions which may undermine her confidence.

This situation provides for doctors and nurses a great opportunity for expanding their traditional roles. To use it they need to understand mother and child as a unit, to utilize the mother's qualities for the recovery of the patient, to give her support in times of stress. To be all day with her sick child is stressful for a mother and she will need the care and support of the staff (10, 26, 40, 48).

(c) The objection that young children are more difficult to manage in the presence of the mother has much truth in it, but the criterion of a child's well-being is not his docility —his readiness to submit to examination or hurt by strangers. It is true that he will probably be less submissive in the presence of his mother, but in the long run it is vastly better for him to feel free to protest in her presence than to be quietly submissive in her absence (21, 33).

A related objection raised is that mothers will be 'hysterical' and obstructive if involved in situations that are painful and distressing for their young children. No doubt there are mothers who, no matter how well they are dealt with, are unable to face a painful situation for their child and will try unreasonably to interfere or will run away from it. But, to repeat an earlier statement, it is our experience that the ordinary mother has greater resources of courage than is sometimes believed and that if given the right conditions she will not only wish to stay by her child in moments of hurt and fright but will do so with composure. If brought into the situation in a positive way, supported in her intuition that her very presence is helpful to her child, the ordinary mother will be able to help her child through such difficult experiences. It will, of course, not always be pleasant for the mother, but it is no part of the concept here described to shield mother from distress—it is rather to give her a positive role in a situation which needs her.

There is, however, no simple answer to the question to what extent resident mothers should be present during painful investigations and treatments. It is common enough practice to have the mother hold her child for an injection or during pre-medication, less common for her to be present during the induction of anaesthesia or immediately after the operation. And she is often excluded from the removal of burn dressings.

Sometimes when a doctor decides that a mother should be excluded from a procedure on grounds that it will distress her to see her child hurt, closer self-examination may enable him to say that deep down he is just as afraid of the distress he himself would feel to have to hurt the child in the presence of the mother. On the other hand, a mother told that her child is to have a burn dressing removed which will take 'just a minute' may be tempted because of her own fears to accept the implication that she should stay out—yet if encouraged to come in find that she has the strength to do so, and if so be later exceedingly glad that she did.

There is probably no disagreement that if the mother is present and in control of her actions it is infinitely better for the child than the terrifying sense that she has abandoned him to assault and hurt. How far this recommendation can be implemented will depend on the individual training and capacities of the doctor and nurse and the situation they can create, and of course on the particular mother. In a matter so difficult no staff member or mother can be asked to do anything which conflicts with their emotions or understanding. To do so would be to invite mishap. It would therefore be unwise to say categorically that mothers should be present at all procedures. As understanding of its value grows, however, we believe it will be found more and more possible to have the mother present as a positive influence during moments of stress for her child. If a mother is brought into hospital to give her child security, each occasion she is excluded from a treatment or investigation denies the underlying principle—and each proposal to exclude her should therefore give cause for solemn reflection and appraisal.

Having mother in hospital with her sick child is a method of care that has its own problems, not only for the hospital but sometimes also for the family. But these are not always as great as is sometimes anticipated. It is, for instance, sometimes said that mothers with other children would not be able to come into hospital—'And what about father?' It is also sometimes suggested that if the mother goes to hospital with the sick child it will cause undue hardship and even harm to the children left at home.

Experience at Amersham General Hospital (10, 37) shows (and this is surely true of other hospitals) (16, 26, 40) that the great majority of mothers gladly accept the opportunity to come into hospital with their young children and find ways of doing so. Surprisingly, perhaps, since there is a ready assumption that only mothers of first children could come into hospital, most of them have other children. Some give as part reason for their eagerness to accompany their sick child that they have had experience of the disturbing effects on another of their children of having been in hospital when young.

Most fathers too are found to be much in favour of the arrangement, although it deprives them of the company of their wives and may give them a lot of housework to do. Although they are not as intimately concerned with the care of the young child, they are intuitively convinced of the advantages to both child and mother. It is also found that relatives and neighbours are sympathetic and ready to help.

As to the fear that the absence of mother may cause undue hardship and even harm to the children left at home, it has first to be noted that commonly the child of under two, and quite often the under-four, is the youngest child and therefore the one most needing his mother's care. The fact that he is ill or about to undergo operation makes his need of her the greater. The older children, left in familiar surroundings and with father and relatives to care for them, will certainly miss their mother—but not at all to the extent that the younger, less mature, and sick child would if mother were not with him in hospital. His is generally by far the greatest need, and therefore he has the greatest claim on her.

If the hospital arrangement is permissive it may be possible for the mother to maintain effective contact with the children at home while devoting most of her attention to the one who is sick. Many expedients have been observed—mothers who slip home for an hour while the patient is asleep and a nurse is standing by; fathers who get up very early and relieve mother before going to work so that she can hurry home and give the other children breakfast and a warm send-off to school, with father coming in again in the evening from work so that mother can be home for an hour at the other children's bedtime; fathers who bring the other children into the hospital grounds where they can meet their mother; big sisters who deputize for mother for an afternoon.

These and other expedients can make it possible for a family to get through a critical time, for the little child who is sick to be kept secure and comforted in hospital and the others not to be neglected. The mother may have to exert herself to the limit to cope with her divided family; but most mothers are so motivated that they would not wish it otherwise, and it is a wise doctor or ward nurse who is content to help them find their own solutions.

It can happen, of course, that the patient is not the youngest, that there is a still younger child at home who may react adversely to the absence of the mother. The only adequate solution to this situation may seem revolutionary. It is that this child too should be in close touch with his mother, possibly by giving him a cot in an adjacent or nearby room.

Otherwise, if there is a child younger than the patient and he cannot stay with his mother, hospital and family must resort to expedients to maintain next best contact. It might be possible, for instance, to have the smaller one much of the day on the hospital lawn or in a playroom where mother could be with him; the nurses, incidentally, would have useful experience of a healthy child.

Not every mother presses to be admitted to hospital with her young child, or accepts immediately she is invited to do so. The maternal impulse to stay with the young child in illness is sometimes overlaid by fear of the hospital situation, or by submission to the traditional practice of giving the sick child over entirely to the hospital. But if given encouragement and reassurance these mothers will generally shed their initial reluctance and prove to be as concerned and adequate as those whose response is more immediate.

The fear is sometimes expressed that if mothers come into hospital to help in the care of their children the nurse will lose an important part of her function and training—the care of young children. In practice this appears to be unjustified; in fact the role of the nurse is enriched and not diminished. Mothers-in does not exclude the nurse, who still carries responsibility on behalf of the hospital and is therefore in constant contact with both child and mother—doing the technical nursing, keeping a discreet eye on the situation, and generally by word and deed helping the mother through the strenuous experience of being all the time with her sick child. The skill of the nurse extends to include mother and child as an entity, and there is much here that is new to learn. And there are always young children whose mothers for some reason are unable to come into hospital and who therefore need full staff care. Although the proposition that mothers should help in the care of their own children may create anxiety among those who have experience only of traditional methods of ward management, it seems that the staffs of mothers-in units prefer the system to the old (26).

Many of the considerations discussed above are illustrated in two complementary publications.

(a) The film *Going to Hospital with Mother* (10), in which it will be seen that when the mother of Sally, aged twenty months, comes with her into hospital she continues in her natural maternal function of tending and comforting, and that her presence keeps the child secure. Mother is present during examinations, premedication, and immediately after the operation. With the unobtrusive support of the ward sister and medical staff she is completely adequate although under strain.

The child is appropriately upset by examinations and procedures, but she quickly recovers and at no time shows any of the fretfulness or quiet withdrawal so commonly seen in unaccompanied children. On the fifth day, when she has fully recovered from the operation and is about to be discharged, she is as bright and mischievous as at home— and in a general state of good-humoured well-being which is *never* seen in unaccompanied children of this age on the fifth day in hospital.

There are half a dozen mothers resident in the ward, and although the children of all of them are ill—some seriously—the morale of the mothers is high. It is high because they are able to help in the care of their children, can give each other friendly support, and can work together doing odd jobs for the ward. They live in simple but adequate accommodation improvised in a ward that was not built for the purpose.

(It should be added that when Sally returned home after five days in hospital she showed no fear of separation or other disturbed behaviour of the kind almost invariably seen in young children who have been in hospital without their mothers.)

(*b*) A paper, 'A Mother's Observations on the Tonsillectomy of Her Four-Year-Old Daughter' (11), in which a mother gives a detailed account of the behaviour of her child before, during, and after an operation, and how she prepared the child for the experience and helped her work through it in hospital and afterwards. Among other things the paper shows clearly how much anxiety the prospect of surgery can create for a child, and how the presence and understanding of the mother can help the child keep her anxiety under control.

A unit for mothers and children will not be successful unless the staff are persuaded of its value, believe that mother is the best person for the child, and regard her not as a rival and a complication but as part of the patient's treatment. An example of this has been observed in the private wing of a hospital in which children in the general wards could be visited twice a week only. In the private wing mothers could stay in separate rooms with their children, and have such refinements as television and record-players. But they were not encouraged to take responsibility and care for their children. Nurses brought them meals and made their beds, and resented 'being waitresses to the mothers'. The mothers, on the other hand, undoubtedly felt that since they were paying high prices for the privilege of being with their children they were entitled to whatever services the ward provided and naturally accepted the role of guest that was given them. They sat around in good clothes, ornamenting their rooms, being attended by the nurses—and feeling bored.

The result was a constant undercurrent of tension between staff and mothers for which neither was responsible, and which could have been relieved had it been understood explicitly that mother's proper role was to minister to the general comfort of her child. Instead of that the arrangement was understood only in financial terms by the hospital, and as an imposition by the nurses. As an example of the tension this created, it was noticed that although the nurses resented having to attend to both child and mother they would nevertheless paradoxically obstruct a mother who tried to do quite small things for her child.

Therefore the mothers could only sit in the rooms all day, reading or watching television, not daring to give their child such simple care as potting or washing. The very fact of the mother's presence was still of great value to the children in that private wing, but the possibility of it being a still greater satisfaction to mother, child, and staff had not been realized.

Finally, it should be said that the workings of the few mothers-in units of which we have first-hand experience are not yet based firmly on the mental health principle that having mothers-in is not just to make children less miserable while in hospital, but to protect their social and emotional development. As previously stated, this principle of mental health has as much validity as the principles of asepsis have for physical health. When the mental health principle is accepted, all the knowledge on which it is based and all the implications that derive from it will become part of the training and practice of the hospital professions. Argument will cease and a new level of organization and procedures will have been achieved.

At present we are far removed from that stage. The wards known to me are well-run, and the mothers and children admitted to them are indeed fortunate. But generally the success of the provision turns on the unusual qualities of some individual—for example a ward sister with special insight into families and no rivalry with mothers—or upon a chance grouping of like-minded people, a consultant, a ward sister, an unusual registrar. This is a precarious basis for work of such importance, because if the ward sister leaves or a new registrar is appointed who is temperamentally opposed to what has been done the whole arrangement could immediately come to an end and the ward revert to traditional practice.

What is now needed is a fuller acceptance into medical and nursing training of the established knowledge of mental health that is now available, so that such empirical humanistic work becomes consolidated in a body of sound knowledge and is no longer dependent on exceptional people. Then the mental health provisions that we advocate will be implemented as routine, just as now the principles of asepsis are routinely applied.

VISITING AND SYSTEMS OF NURSING

If the mother is for any reason unable to stay with her young child in hospital, it is necessary to discover the next best ways of implementing the concept that he needs 'a warm, intimate, and continuous relationship to the mother, or to one permanent mother-substitute'. Two related aspects have to be considered: *Visiting by the Parents* and *Systems of Nursing*.

Visiting (a) Some General Considerations

The next best thing to the mother being in hospital with her child is of course unrestricted visits by the mother, during which she tends him as she would do at home.

The classical opposition to visiting has been on grounds that when young children have 'settled' they are made unhappy by the visits of their parents. But, as has been discussed earlier, it is a fallacy that 'settled' young children are 'happy' in any reasonable meaning of that term; the parental visit merely releases feelings of grief and anger that had been concealed. Furthermore, it is now proven by the experience of many wards that if visiting arrangements are liberalized the amount of severe crying diminishes—at least among the three- and four-year-olds—and that parents too are less agitated.

But although many wards have reached the stage of daily visiting and have come to appreciate its benefits, they hesitate to take the next step of removing all restrictions on visiting. They fear the consequence would be that they would be overrun by mothers who would stay all day and that the work of the ward would be impeded. Here again the experience of those wards which have initiated unrestricted visiting should allay anxiety. They are not overrun and work is not impeded, although some aspects of the work may need to be rearranged. The consultant may find that it is discreet to discuss patients with his juniors in the duty room before going on a ward round, instead of in a ward with parents present; this has the incidental advantage that the young patient does not hear remarks that he can misconstrue. If the consultant stops expecting that parents be excluded from the ward while he and his party make the round he will probably find that he is met with more respect and less obsequiousness, and that mother and child are more interesting together than apart—for him and students alike. Staff and parents will have much more respect for and appreciation of each other. And all in all the ward will be a livelier, though perhaps less tidy, place.

To tell parents that they may visit at any time is a more positive and more revolutionary step than may at first appear. It is not merely a matter of opening the ward to visitors. Just as significantly it says to the parent, '*You* decide when you will come and how long you will stay. *You* know best what this child needs from you, and how you should distribute your time between him and those at home.'

This attitude is of course almost that of the well-run mothers-in unit mentioned above, and is surely only a step short of it in practice. It respects the mother as the most important person for her child and as a person of good intuitive judgement—not as an irritating appendage of the patient. It does not say any more, 'Come at this time or that, and an hour a day at teatime is best—we know better than you'.

Left to do as they wish in this way it is found that mothers will often spend lengthy parts of the first days with the sick child, leaving him only when he is tucked down for the night; then if the child is old enough to understand and well enough to allow her to do so (particularly if he can be transferred to a single nurse) mother will gradually cut down on the time spent in the ward and give more attention to her duties elsewhere. It is most important to realize that in this matter the mother is allowed to be herself, supported and advised if necessary by the staff but not directed.

Some Implications for Hospital Practice

The less restricted the visiting, the more relaxed become the relationships between staff and parents. There is less wielding of authority, and mothers take over many of the simple tasks of care for their children—feeding, potting, washing, brushing hair. Apart from the incidental help this is to the work of the ward, its value to the child is immense. The young child knows much of his mother's love through her handling of his body, and if she can be there and tend him in this maternal way much has been done for his comfort and security.

However, unrestricted visiting, like any kind of visiting, is more successful with older children than with younger. For any child of three years and under it will be distressing when the mother leaves the ward each day—no matter how many hours she has spent with him. Such is the nature of his dependency on her. The three- or four-year-old will also show distress but will usually have enough intellectual maturity and time-sense to understand that mother will come next day. The inability of the younger child to accept explanations or to tolerate frustration merely emphasizes that although unrestricted visiting is a great and welcome advance it still falls short of the needs of the younger ones.

Most wards, of course, do not have unrestricted visiting and may well not accept the desirability or practicability of it. Visiting for an hour a day may be the most that can be achieved in the immediate future. If so, some of the points already made have to be borne in mind—that these visiting parents may be less reliable and less well related to the staff than those who can visit freely, and that there will be more distress in the under-fours than if they had more of their mothers.

It is then vital to bear in mind that if a young patient

cries during and after a visit it is not usually the direct result of the visit. It is natural that the child should cry for his mother. It is not that her visit makes him unhappy, but simply that it causes his feelings to break through into tears. The painful separation is beyond his understanding, and he not only longs for his mother but is angry that she abandons him between visits. It may sometimes seem that a two- or three-year-old derives little benefit from a visit. But the visits do help him in at least two ways—by discharging some of the feeling that might otherwise remain pent up inside, and by giving him some reassurance that his parents still exist and care for him. Otherwise there would be no gleam of hope in his desolation.

An obstacle to accepting that it is normal and appropriate for the young child to be so distressed is the fiction—not yet totally discredited—that children's wards are happy places. Certainly, if an older child is tended with consideration the nurses will be rewarded for their efforts by his being cheerful and contented. But nothing can compensate the younger child for the absence of his mother, and his unresponsive misery is not rewarding for the nurse who would like him to be as cheerful and contented as the older ones. The nurse who understands the simple fact that young children are in this respect so different from the older ones does not try to 'cheer-up' the tearful little one while avoiding reference to the reason for his grief. She shows sympathetic understanding of his feelings, makes it clear that she knows he wants his mother, and comforts him in his tears. In this way she helps him immeasurably more than by trying to jolly him out of his distress.

As long as visits to the young child are restricted, the problem of how to give him as much security and reassurance as possible between times remains. Its solution can be approached in many ways—for example, by allowing him to bring his favourite 'cuddly' or toy (if he has such) to hospital and making absolutely sure that this strong emotional link with home is not taken away no matter how dilapidated it becomes; by giving him something to keep that he knows mother values and will certainly return to claim, such as a glove or small purse; by sending regular postcards which a nurse will be sure to read and explain as often as he asks, and which he can keep in his cot.

At the end of visiting time it is important that if the child is old enough to have any understanding he should be told truthfully that his parents are going but will come again—*never* that they are going 'just for a moment'; and that they know he wants to come home—they too want him home and he will come home as soon as the hospital say he is better. It is also very helpful if a nurse he knows stands by to comfort him when his parents have gone (14, 20, 23, 27, 38, 43, 49).

But in relation to the young child's need even daily contact for an hour is pitifully small. For the schoolchild of, say, 8 plus, who can understand the situation and has already achieved considerable emotional independence from his parents, who can read and write and talk with people to occupy himself, the daily visit is usually quite adequate and a spell in hospital no great hardship. But for the younger ones who are wholly parent-oriented brief daily visits touch no more than the fringe of their needs. The fact that a two-year-old 'settles down' under daily visiting is no more evidence of his well-being than the fact that he 'settles down' under weekly visiting. If daily visiting were adequate the children would not show distress during visits and afterwards, and would not be disturbed in their behaviour when they return home. But they *do* show distress, and they *are* disturbed in their later behaviour.

A current tendency to regard daily visiting as a panacea and the goal of reform is therefore ill-founded. Advance though it is, daily visiting is still inadequate for younger children and their parents and is associated with much stress (23). The study by Prugh *et al.* (44) already referred to on page 7 showed that although better ward management including daily visiting considerably reduced the incidence of disturbance in a group of children aged from 2 to 10 years, this improvement was much less in the younger children than in the older—in fact it was principally the younger children who continued to show disturbance.

Visiting   (b) *In Fever Hospitals*

In many British fever (isolation) hospitals patients are not allowed to be visited, the reason given being that the risk to the visitor and to the community of conveyed infection is too great. Although a discussion of the medical aspects does not come within the scope of this book, it does appear that if the staff of a fever hospital believe visiting to be of value they will find ways of making it possible.

In a number of American hospitals there has been daily visiting in infectious wards for some years. A statement by the medical superintendent of an Australian hospital, made five years ago, is quite explicit and may be quoted in full:

'It has long been realized that the isolation of patients has had little effect on the control of epidemics and it appeared that the separation of patients from all contact with relatives during the infectious period is an unnecessary hardship which can be shown to react in some cases unfavourably on the patients' progress.

'We have limited the number of visitors to any one patient at a time to two close relatives. We also issue the following instructions to each visitor—

1. Do not go in to patient until given permission by a member of nursing staff.
2. *Wear a gown whilst at the bedside.* In certain cases a mask will also be worn, covering nose and mouth.
3. Avoid close contact with patient, and do *not* visit when suffering from cold or sore throat.
4. At end of visit wash hands with soap and running water, remove gown, hang it on back of chair in wards, and then rinse hands a second time.
5. The mother of a child patient may be given opportunity to assist the nurse in preparing the child for sleep during evening visiting. This may *only* be done with the nurse present.
6. Food, fruit, or sweets, may not be given to children. Parcels with child's name on, to be left at entrance to ward.
7. Cot sides must not be let down.

'The innovation to date has been so successful that it would be most unlikely that we would revert to the old system. Daily visiting by relatives has improved the morale of all fever patients both adults and children. The improvement in the general public relations of the hospital has been shown by the tone of the letters of thanks received from the relatives. The old attitude of suspicion as to what goes on in a fever hospital has been largely removed by the daily personal contact with the nursing staff and with the ward doctor. The nursing and medical staff also have received valuable training in the tactful handling of relatives, often a neglected art in public hospitals. The older members of the nursing staff have accepted the change and have been quick to appreciate the advantages in the management of the patient. Many valuable suggestions originating from the staff have been incorporated in the scheme and have assisted in the organization.

'As part of the scheme, encouragement is given to mothers of difficult children either to live in hospital for a few days or else to attend at mealtimes and so provide help to busy nurses who otherwise may waste valuable nursing hours in procedures which can often be more simply done by the mother.

'Since the commencement of daily visiting in the infectious wards there has not been one complaint from any relative or from the outside public that visiting has been responsible for transmission of infection to outside sources. I would be surprised if there had been any trouble, but all care is taken to see that there are no grounds for criticism. The visitors must take the same precautions as doctors and nurses; and if this is done it should be sufficient answer to any complaint' (18).

Experiments along these lines have been successfully made in some British fever hospitals (37). The importance which ordinary parents attach to such provisions was specially clearly shown in our first-hand experience.

The five-year-old daughter of a working-class couple got scarlet fever and was admitted to an isolation hospital in the London area. Her parents promised the child that they would visit her each day, but were told in the admission room that visiting was not allowed and that they could collect their daughter in three weeks' time. The favourite toy which they had thoughtfully brought with the child to help maintain the link with home was returned to them with the remark that the hospital could provide all the toys the child needed. On the way out they peeped into the ward and saw their child lying sobbing.

The parents were understandably most unhappy, not only that they would not see their child for so long but because they knew she would feel they had let her down. Later that day they heard of a fever hospital in another part of London which was experimenting with daily visiting, and made such firm representations to the medical superintendent of the first hospital (who told them they were just 'fussy') that the child was transferred by ambulance to the hospital in which she could be visited.

As is implied in the Australian statement given above, such opposition to visiting by parents as is based on the argument that they might contract infectious diseases or convey them into the community is not entirely reasonable. Porters, radiographers, and ward maids as well as doctors and nurses go into isolation wards and also move freely in the community. Isolation hospitals which permit visiting simply ensure that parents observe the same precautions as staff.

Isolation hospitals tend to be more shut off from the community and from progressive ideas than other hospitals. This can be reflected both in resistance to visiting and in less enlightened handling of children in their wards.

Systems of Nursing

The less contact the young patient has with his mother, whether because she cannot or is not allowed to be with him, the more important does the system of nursing become. For instance, if mother is with him all or most of the time, it is of little account whether one or more nurses are involved. But if mother is there for only an hour or so a day it is of the greatest importance how his nursing is provided during the other twenty-three.

In most hospitals he will be dealt with by a number of nurses during the day, the majority of them students; and because of lectures, the shift system, and movement between wards in course of training, it can readily happen that in the course of a week twenty nurses will have shared in his care. Each of them may be kindly, but such fragmented attention does not meet his primary need of mothering, and he is confused by more people than his limited capacity can comprehend. The nursing of children should be by 'case assignment' and not by 'work assignment' or the 'team' methods which are now general. The main features of these systems are as follows.

Work or Job Assignment: the traditional method of organizing nursing and still the method most commonly in use. Duties are so arranged that the senior nurses do the treatments and investigations and the juniors mainly the more domestic and routine work. A fixed set of duties is prepared for each nurse, either according to seniority or on a rota basis. This means that all the nurses attend to some part of the nursing care of each patient. The care of the child is thus fragmented among a number of people so that although his bodily needs may be efficiently met his emotional needs are not (30).

Team or Group Assignment: the patients are divided into groups, each of which is tended by a number of nurses working as a team. This method brings the nurses into closer and more satisfactory relationship with their patients, and is increasingly advocated and practised. It represents a great advance on the work assignment method, and for adults and older children the method has much to commend it. But for these younger ones it is still short of the optimum nursing provision.

Case Assignment: a number of beds and cots are allocated to each nurse; and the nurse, irrespective of seniority, takes any patient, however ill, admitted to these beds. No matter how senior or junior she is, the nurse does everything for her own patients and is present at all treatments and investigations. The more junior the nurse, of course, the more supervision she requires. The work of the ward is so organized that off-duty times are relieved by a few other nurses only who are also on the ward staff and known to the patients. The benefit of this method to the younger patient is that he has a 'special' nurse whom he knows to be 'his' nurse and with whom he can feel more secure, a nurse who will understand him as an individual because of the variety of things she does for him, and who can pass on information about his characteristics to whoever relieves her for off-duty periods (45).

In case assignment the nurse has in effect a small family of patients for whom she does everything in the way that a mother would, and when she has time off she is relieved by someone who is also familiar to them. This is the system of nursing that best meets the psychological needs of the young child in the absence of the mother, because it gives him a mother substitute. Discovering that she is 'his' nurse and that it is always she who does things for him, he will become attached to her in a way that allows him to give free rein to a range of feelings that would otherwise become frozen. He will act as a normal child as the family acts towards his mother—demanding, affectionate, trusting, and sometimes angry towards his nurse (12). This is a much healthier state of mind to be in than he would otherwise exhibit, but it takes more understanding and management than when he is docile and undemanding.

This consequence of a system of nursing that is immeasurably better for younger children than any other requires understanding from the nurse, and appropriate selection and training. It has also two interesting practical implications—that the nurse should have opportunities for getting skilled advice on the behaviour of individual patients; and that, subject only to such advice and to medical necessity, she should be allowed considerable discretion in the way she handles them. Thus it will be seen that the application of a quite simple concept of child care has larger implications than might appear—in this instance that traditionally strict control over the spontaneity of nurses would require to be relaxed in this 'non-medical' area in the interests of the young patient.

The efficacy of case-assignment nursing will of course be limited by the 48 hour week, or 96 hour fortnight, but careful planning can ensure that a minumum number of nurses relieve each other for time off—so limiting the total number who deal with each child. This is not easily arranged in hospitals that are short of staff, or where the training curricula require that student nurses move to other wards at fixed points in their training. But if meeting the emotional needs of the young patient is understood to be a paramount consideration, both of the child himself and in the training of the student nurse, she will not be moved until her small family have all been discharged home. And if the patients are to be long-stay their nurses should be permanent and not students. (The care of long-stay patients is referred to below.)

Case-assignment nursing is not popular in the nursing profession because it is much more difficult to manage than more traditional methods which are administratively tidier, and because it conflicts with conventional views about the improving status of the student nurse as her training progresses. 'Team or group care', though still less than optimal for the younger patient, is a move in the right direction. But when it becomes sufficiently understood that as much attention has to be given to mental health as to asepsis no considerations of administration or status will be allowed to stand in the way of providing the optimal system of nursing care. The case-assignment role is usually found to have more satisfaction within it for the nurse than any other method.

But a system of nursing can never be so adequate as to justify restricting contact between the young child and his mother. The substitution of a nurse will not prevent the severe stress and potential trauma of an actual separation from the mother, though care by a case-assigned nurse will greatly minimize other risks to his emotional security. Ideally, case-assignment nursing would operate concurrently with maximum access and participation by the mother—thus ensuring that the child's emotional security is maintained at the best possible level and his return to the family accomplished with the least difficulty.

THE SPECIAL PROBLEM OF THE LONG-STAY WARD

In the foregoing discussion of short-term hospitalization the thesis has been that ways should be found to maintain close contact between young patients and their mothers—

preferably by the mother coming into residence or, failing that, visiting without restriction.

The long-stay patient presents a more serious problem of care, though one that for a variety of reasons attracts less attention than that of the short-stay patient. Long-stay wards generally have less visiting than other hospitals, partly because they are more socially structured and isolated communities which fear that the school work of the children would be obstructed if parents could visit at any time, and partly because they tend to be at such distance from the districts they serve that working parents cannot find time or money to visit more often than once or twice weekly.

The argument that more frequent visiting would interfere with education and the work of the ward cannot be taken entirely at its face value. Although the argument has some truth it is also used to rationalize traditional resistance to the presence of parents. It is obviously not true for children under four that their education would be interfered with, and probably not even for children under seven, and no restriction whatever should be placed on the visiting of these children—young enough in years to need their parents, and made still younger by illness and confinement to bed. For children over seven visiting should be restricted only during the few school hours, and even then not rigidly. The overriding consideration should be the emotional needs and mental health of the child of any age.

If parents live at such distance that fares are a serious consideration, travel and subsistence should be available to them easily and without means test. Such is the importance for mental health to be attached to maintaining parent-child links. The matter has already been the subject of a finding in an international conference (28).

Some Implications for Hospital Practice

Sometimes young children are sent to distant hospitals for no better reason than that beds happen to be available, and in disregard of their emotional needs. Every attempt should be made to treat long-stay young patients in hospitals near their homes and to send them home at week-ends and holidays. Whenever it is proposed to send any child, particularly if he is under eight, to a hospital that is not easily accessible to his parents, the question should be asked: cannot this treatment be given locally?

But even if it were provided that mothers could stay with their children in long-stay hospitals, or that they could have fares and subsistence paid for as much visiting as they wished, it would in fact generally be impracticable for a mother to devote herself so completely to her sick child for months or years—though if she could and wished to do so it should be permitted. The danger that threatens the long-stay young patient owing to the loss of mother's care and the infrequency of visiting is that, because of the large number of nurses who will share in his care, he will be deprived over a long period of the conditions necessary for his mental health. If this is accepted, a firm obligation rests upon the hospital to compensate as fully as possible for the loss of maternal care.

'Case-assignment' nursing has already been discussed as the best way of meeting the primary need of the young patient, and a variant of this system is the only answer we know of to the problem of the long-stay child. The permanence of the ward sister or staff nurse does not of itself meet the requirement since their availability spreads too thinly over the ward. And quite obviously student nurses cannot give continuity over months or years. The only solution is that the care of young patients should be done entirely by permanent staff. Student nurses should play no significant part in their care.

This proposal is readily rejected as impractical on grounds that the general shortage of nurses necessitates that the burden of ward work be carried by students, and that students must work in children's wards if they are to learn about children. It cannot be too strongly emphasized however, that an important principle of mental health is at stake and that no practical difficulties should be allowed to prevent its implementation—just as the requirements of asepsis would not be disregarded for any reason.

There would appear to be two alternative ways of providing substitute mothering in long-stay wards. Firstly, permanent nurses only could be employed on 'case assignment', with students as supernumeraries or entirely absent and getting their children's training in short-stay wards; or secondly, a solution that would be much preferable wherever practicable, that the social organization of long-stay wards be radically re-conceived —not as a hospital with teaching and occupation provided, but as a children's home with medical attention provided. The difference in approach is considerable, and if adopted would revolutionize the care of young long-term patients.

There are many long-stay hospitals in which the main part of the care could be given by women who are not nurses but foster-mothers—each acting as mother to a little family group and doing for each child those things which a mother does at home and which she would do in a mothers-in unit. Doctors and nurses would come in only as necessary for medical reasons. The standards of the ward would be those of a children's home, not those of a hospital ward. The management of the children, except in matters strictly determined by medical necessity, would be under a lay head trained in the day-to-day care of children and not in their diseases. The foster-mothers would be answerable to her, and not to the medical and nursing staff. In organization if not in finance and administration it would therefore be a children's home adjacent to appropriate medical facilities.

At present nurses usually do all tasks, from face-washing to special dressings. If in long-stay wards they retained only the technical aspects, and all other care were given by foster-mothers, the child's need of a stable maternal-type relationship would be met—and incidentally the nursing shortage would be relieved. This proposal may well be resisted in the profession as an attack on the function of nurses. To this the answer is surely that the primary concern must be what is best for the long-stay patient.

This proposal for the re-structuring of long-stay hospitals may seem revolutionary but the notion is not new in child care. The fact is that the 'non-medical' care of children in hospitals, particularly in long-stay hospitals, lags far behind modern knowledge and practice in other institutions for children. The Report of the Care of Children Committee (The 'Curtis' Committee) of 1946, which led to the Children Act of 1948, recommended that children who 'for any cause whatever' are deprived of a normal home life with their parents or relatives should be cared for in small family groups so that they could experience the stable relationships and the rich emotional life that the more fortunate child finds in the family. These recommendations initiated a period of radical change in the organization of institutions for healthy children and in the training of their staffs, and during the past ten years it has been increasingly the practice to care for healthy deprived children in small family groups. This is a tremendous advance on the fragmented group care which still characterizes very many children's wards—a method of care which does justice neither to the devoted nurse nor to the child patient.

Unfortunately, the remit to the Curtis Committee did not include consideration of the 'non-medical' care of sick children. But there is no doubt that similar urgent considerations apply. The similarity is perhaps obscured by the fact that most young children in long-stay wards have loving families awaiting their return, so that they are not technically 'deprived'. But their actual experience of deprivation of maternal-type care while in a long-stay ward can be severe, despite the weekly visit and the kind intention of the staff, and despite the deceptive cheerfulness of many of these young patients. There is need for a 'Curtis Committee type' of inquiry into the care of children in hospital, particularly long-stay hospitals (5, 8, 13).

A Note on Play in the Long-Stay Ward

Young children who are confined to cots should not be denied certain pleasurable activities that are available to those who are ambulant and able to go to nursery school. It sometimes happens that cot-bound children are not allowed to play with sand, water, or finger-paints because these might 'mess' the cot sheets or the floor. These objections, when made, usually come from the nursing staff and may be a cause of friction between them and the teaching staff.

All young children pass through a phase of messy play, and in the family this is usually taken for granted and facilitated. For the young patient this messy play is an important therapeutic activity, and should be provided for without regard to the polish on the floor or the whiteness of the sheets. Of course, in a long-stay ward conceived as a children's home, as suggested on p. 66, in charge of lay people and with medical and technical nursing attention provided as extras, there would be no difficulty about making such provisions. The standards of the ward would be those of a children's home, and a potential source of frustration to child and teacher would be removed.

PREPARATION OF THE YOUNG CHILD FOR HOSPITAL

The preparation of a child for going to hospital is a difficult subject on which we shall not elaborate because of the complex variables that enter in—such as age, reason for hospitalization, amount of contact to be allowed, temperament of parents. But some basic points can be made.

The problem is again one of age and maturity. The older the child the more likely it is that he can be prepared; the younger he is, the less likely. It should, for instance, be possible to discuss the necessity for hospitalization with a child of 8 or 10 plus and get his full acceptance and cooperation; and the experience, unless very prolonged and associated with unusual degrees of illness and pain, should cause little disturbance to him. But as we go down the age scale it becomes increasingly difficult to prepare, and ultimately *impossible*, because of immaturity, lack of understanding of the environment, and lack of verbal understanding.

For the child old enough to be helped in this way, preparation is likely to be more successful if done by the parents and if associated with truthful assurance that they will remain in contact with him and fetch him home again as soon as he is well. (The task is much more difficult if the child is going to a long-stay hospital with only weekly visiting, or into one of the isolation hospitals which allow none.)

He (or she) should be told simply and truthfully *why* he has to go to hospital. Young children get strange ideas about the reasons for things. Not uncommonly when they go to hospital they feel they are being punished or sent away for ever because they have been naughty, and if they are not given the true reason for going to hospital this is the kind of frightening reason they are likely to invent.

He should, if possible, be given a general impression of what being in hospital is like, so that it will not seem totally strange when he gets there—for instance, that children are in bed and have dinner and tea there; that he may have to use a pot instead of going to the toilet; that doctors and nurses dress in white and sometimes wear masks. (There are now useful leaflets to be had with drawings of ward scenes on which these unfamiliar aspects of ward life can be pointed out (14).)

No pretence should be made that the experience will be fun, like going to a party or having ice-cream. It is tempting to say nothing to him about the unpleasant things—like pain and anaesthetics—but it is not helpful to ignore them. If he has to meet pain and discomfort it will be much less disturbing for him if he has an inkling about them beforehand. Therefore, if he is to have an operation he should be told in a simple matter-of-fact way, preferably some days beforehand, so that he has time to ask questions and to get reassurance.

He should be told that he will have 'a special sleep' and will wake up again in a little while. And that he will probably not feel very well—and that it will hurt a little. But *that it will be getting better all the time.*

It would be neither possible nor desirable to anticipate everything that might happen to him in hospital, such as injections, enemas, and other incidental procedures. Advance notice of these might cause an unnecessary degree of apprehension. All he needs are a few signposts to assure him that what happens is according to plan, *and that his mother knows about it*. Incidental treatments and investigations are best intimated to him immediately before they occur, preferably by his mother but otherwise by his own nurse.

It is better that he is not told too far ahead that he is going to hospital; otherwise the lengthy waiting may build up undue anxiety. Nor should explanations be given him in one go. Best of all, if it can be achieved, is to begin telling him about a week in advance—telling him a little and then expanding at the pace set by his questions. Thus the repetitions he needs can be given as he needs them, and all the information necessary given in the order in which he can best assimilate it. (Sometimes, unfortunately, good intention is defeated by mishap, as when the child overhears the doctor recommend his admission to hospital and by showing anxiety about the prospect compels his parents to talk about it weeks ahead. In that event it is better to tell the child what he wants to know than to try to ignore his anxieties (11).)

I believe it to be completely mistaken to think that children of under four or five can be reassured by seeing the ward and its apparatus before admission. But if it is known that the anaesthetic will be administered by mask while the child is still conscious, some playful demonstration of this could be given by the mother.

In letting the child help pack to go to hospital it can be useful to let him see also the preparations for his return—that his clean clothes are being got ready, for instance—as an additional assurance that he will be coming home again.

71

Young Children in Hospital

But still lower down the age scale preparation is increasingly difficult, or impossible. The child of 2½ or 3 may seem to understand that mother is going to leave him, but this is in fact a concept the real nature of which he is incapable of appreciating. Since mother is so much part of him he cannot truly imagine life without her; so that, even if he seems to understand, the first experience of being in hospital and out of her care overwhelms him and any glimmering of understanding is swept away.

Some slight but helpful notion that going away also means coming back can be given in non-verbal ways to a child of this age by playing little games in which mother goes away (out of the room) *and comes back*, or teddy bear is sent 'to hospital' and warmly welcomed home again. But the inescapable fact is that in this age group little can be done to make loss of the mother comprehensible and tolerable. The moral is again that these children are too young to be away from their mothers, and that attention should be given not to the unrewarding task of 'preparing' them but to finding ways of maintaining maximum contact between the child and his mother.

Personal Toys and Possessions

Many young children have a toy or other object—for instance a teddy bear, rag doll, piece of eiderdown—which constant handling has rendered almost unrecognizable. They derive much satisfaction from a possession brought with them through earlier stages of development and will cling to it especially when tired or unwell (55).

It is of the utmost importance that if a young child has such a prized object it should accompany him to hospital.

There it will give him comfort, and make a link with home and all the love and care that are there. It will give some security when the situation is strange and perhaps frightening. Parents may need help in understanding this, and have to be discouraged from trying to substitute an expensive plaything. A new toy is no substitute for the prized object, no matter how disreputable it may appear to the adult eye. Student nurses too should be taught to be vigilant in ensuring that the favoured toy or 'cuddly' does not go astray (6).

A young child may have a special way of getting off to sleep. He may clutch or finger a piece of soft material, something with a texture whose 'feel' brings a sense of contentment that is linked to an earlier stage in his development and that is so specific to him that no other texture will take its place. This going-to-sleep habit is everywhere known to parents, and everywhere respected. Therefore, if a little child has such a comfort habit he should take the 'thing' with him to hospital and it should be an important part of his nursing care to ensure that the 'thing' is always within his reach. It may be necessary to caution the student nurse that an apparently useless scrap of material is of great consolation to him. Otherwise her wish to tidy the cot may deprive him of it.

Sometimes a young child will come to hospital with a 'dummy' ('pacifier' in America). Staff should think twice before depriving a child of a 'dummy', even if he appears too old for one. For some children this is just another means of finding comfort, and it should be respected. In the situation of being ill and away from home he can well be allowed this consolation, especially if his parents have not thought it necessary to deprive him of it (10).

Young Children in Hospital

Guidance for Parents on Preparation

There is a variety of books and leaflets intended to help parents prepare children for going to hospital, some good and some not so good. The great defect in many of them is that although the intention is to help the child through a difficult experience they avoid or minimize three main aspects of the problem:

(a) That the child if young will be unhappy, and that there will be other crying children in the ward.

(b) That there will be pain after operation.

(c) That on return home the child will be difficult in his behaviour.

Such publications are half-hearted and therefore only half-helpful about the problem. If parents understand that their young child will probably cry when they visit and be awkward for a time after return home they will know that it is normal and not a defect in themselves or the child. But unfortunately the authors of some leaflets appear unwilling to acknowledge that hospital can be so upsetting.

On a more ambitious level there are books which children can read or paint. They can be most useful, though again more in the upper age range, but commonly show three serious shortcomings:

(a) Everyone is shown smiling all the time—doctors, nurses, parents, and patients.

(b) There is too much representation of frightening procedures of a kind that are best intimated to the child when they are about to be done—e.g. injections. To show them graphically in a preparatory book can build up considerable and unnecessary anticipatory anxiety.

(c) The child who is too young to be helped by words or pictures is totally ignored, not even acknowledged as the significant exception.

Some Implications for Hospital Practice

Among the better books which are content to familiarize the child with the features of general ward activity that will be strange to him is *Going to the Hospital* (15). A modest leaflet that is recommended, *Coming Into Hospital* (14), presents guidance to parents in simple terms that they can use with little modification in talking to their child. It also provides an outline drawing of a children's ward scene containing a variety of ward situations—a useful device in presenting ideas to the small child whose capacity for verbal understanding is limited. This leaflet acknowledges, as too few others do, that the young child will inevitably be distressed by being in hospital, that the younger he is the less possible it is to prepare him, and that whatever is attempted should therefore be supported by as much visiting by the mother as is allowed.

However, useful though leaflets and books are, there are many parents who are unable to make effective use of them because of their own anxiety about the impending hospitalization. Such parents may tell their children about hospital in a misleading way, or shirk it altogether. It would be especially valuable if hospitals were to regard leaflets as only part of the help needed by parents. It would be helpful if, a week or so before the child's admission, the parents were interviewed, either singly or in a group, and the material of the leaflet discussed with them. A good almoner, the right kind of ward sister or paediatrician, a psychiatric social worker or psychologist from the clinic, would help greatly by dealing in this way with some of the parental anxieties. The time given would be well spent (53).

75

Young Children in Hospital

More attention should be given to the effect on parents of their child being sent to hospital. As far as is known no studies have been done, but from general experience some comments can be made.

Parents are glad that there are hospitals with all the resources of skill and equipment for restoring their child to health, but if the child is young they are rightly upset by the necessity for hospitalization. They know the child needs love and security and reassurance which only they can properly give, and if he has to go to hospital without his mother they know very well the distress that will ensue (20, 23, 30, 31).

Parents sometimes feel badly about this situation in rather unexpected ways. Although they may intellectually understand the inevitability of hospitalization, they can also feel that they have let the child down by exposing him to stress. If the mother has nursed the child at home up to the point where hospital becomes necessary, and then is shut out from participation in his care, she can and often does feel inadequate in face of the omnipotent and infallible hospital—and, though unreasonably, feel that she has somehow failed as a mother. The doctors and nurses can make her child well when she could not, and they do not allow her any part of his care.

It can happen then that a mother begins to have an unrealistic view of her child, longs so much to have him back in her embrace that she remembers only his lovable qualities and forgets all the exasperating features that he has in common with other children. When he returns and does not fit her fantasy of an angel child who reciprocates her tender feeling, but instead is anxious and aggressive and set back in his toilet training, it can be a blow to her

76

self-esteem. She can readily misinterpret what has happened. Having seen that in hospital he was 'settled' and docile with the nurses, and now finding him difficult to manage, she can feel that she is less good with her child than the nurses were—not realizing that he is now re-acting to the separation experience and not to any fault in her. Many mothers find this embarrassing and humili-ating, and will hardly talk about it. Furthermore they can feel so disappointed that the child has not returned as the cuddly and loving thing they longed for that they may become irritated and be less able than they might have been to be patient with his disturbed behaviour. The mother's self-confidence and self-esteem have been diminished.

This is an additional reason why there should be maximum contact between mother and child, preferably with mother helping in his care. She will remain realistic about his illness and will not get wrong ideas about the kind of child he is. Her confidence in her own worth is sustained. The child, too, will go home with a mother who has stayed by him and coped with his anxieties and kept them from multiplying, instead of going home to a mother on whom he can for the first time unload his feelings of insecurity and anger.

Furthermore the transition from hospital to home will be undramatic. Mother will take over a child whose diets and other requirements she understands because she has participated in their preparation. She will not be faced suddenly by new and perhaps unfamiliar demands on her competence (10, 25, 26). There is a strikingly low incidence of disturbance following hospitalization with the mother (26).

THE REASSESSMENT OF HOSPITAL PROCEDURES

The maintenance of close contact between mother and child, whether by mother-in arrangements or unrestricted visiting, should be supported by procedures and routines reassessed in the light of modern knowledge and conditions. In hospitals, as in all long-established institutions, routines sometimes persist for traditional reasons when the necessity for them has gone. Only constant vigilance based on the wish to minimize anxiety in the child will ensure that the effects of desirable innovations are not vitiated by the persistence of unfavourable and well-established procedures.

Some of the more obvious examples of these have been mentioned above—such as the inconsistency of permitting daily visiting yet prohibiting visiting for the first two days to let the child 'settle'; allowing visiting but not allowing mother to do things for the child; giving parents a leaflet to help them prepare the child for hospital, but failing to ensure that if a favourite toy or cuddly is brought to the hospital it is not lost or removed.

Fifty years ago, when social conditions were much worse than now and the population less clean, it was presumably necessary to put every new admission into a bath. Conditions have changed, and many hospitals now recognize that young patients are usually scrubbed clean before arrival so that it is not necessary to bath them straight away. They go into the ward and play around before being put to bed. Or if exceptionally they do happen to be dirty they are bathed by the mother or in her presence.

In either instance the child is spared the shock of being divested of his clothes and bathed by a stranger. But not every hospital has yet seen the anachronism of the admission bath. Sometimes the kindest of nurses can be the executant of harsh and unnecessary procedures, as seen for instance in the film *A Two-Year-Old Goes to Hospital* (6), in which an excellent and competent mother is left in the waiting-room while a smiling young nurse forces the clothes off a perfectly clean child and bathes her— then goes through the routines of checking pulse and temperature before allowing the sobbing and bewildered child to see her mother again.

In that instance it was, naturally, not the nurse who was at fault. The difficulty arose from the rigid and anachronistic routine from which she could not deviate, a position to which in fact she was forced to conform with the unquestioning obedience of one under a discipline built up for quite different reasons and in a different situation. Obviously, the more humane and reasonable procedure would have been to have mother accompany the child through a minimum of necessary procedures and to stay with the child for some hours at least. But such is force of custom and tradition that the staff had become unaware of the unkindness of the procedure, although it is most evident when seen on film. That is an example of traditional and out-dated procedure which can be revised without harm but will be revised only by conscious effort (52).

Since the prevention of anxiety in the child is the aim, the most important single improvement is to have mother with the child throughout—or, if not mother, then one nurse whom the child will come to know as his special nurse. The initiation into hospital can be immeasurably eased if the mother is there and/or if the nurse who will be responsible for the child begins her duties in the admission room. This nurse should conduct the child and the mother through all reception procedures. And, whether or not the mother stays, this nurse should be present at all significant moments.

No treatment or investigation should be done to the child except in the presence of the mother or special nurse, and the less the mother is able to participate the more essential it is that there should be this special nurse on whom the child can depend. Even apparently minor details such as moving the child from one ward to another, or from open ward into a cubicle, need to be thought of in these terms. The young patient, precariously adapted to a strange new environment, can be terrified by such a move. Many a child has feared that his mother will not find him again if he is not in the place where she last saw him. For these reasons he should not be moved without the assurance that his mother or special nurse, accompanying him during the change, knows where he is. The same applies to young patients sent from hospital for convalescence. This precaution, combined with explanation given by mother or nurse to dispose of the misconstructions that young children constantly place on experiences, can prevent the building up of anxiety to the point where it is overwhelming and potentially damaging.

There is so much evidence of inconsistent practice both between and within hospitals where the wearing of masks by nurses is concerned that the matter might usefully be examined. Children are often frightened by these masks, and it may be that they are sometimes worn more often than is necessary.

Two provisions that are increasingly advocated with the kindly intention of making young patients 'happy' need comment:

Some Implications for Hospital Practice

(*a*) In some wards it is encouraged that no professional member of staff—nurse, social worker, medical student, doctor, anaesthetist—should go through the ward without sparing time to pick up a child and say a friendly word. The intention is laudable, but it is mistaken for reasons already given at length. The young child needs love from the one or two persons he knows. To be handled, however kindly, by a variety of people does not help at all but merely confuses the child—and may prevent the staff from giving full attention to the basic problem.

(*b*) It is sometimes advocated that 'volunteers', namely men and women from the community who have time and interest, should be organized to provide recreation for and affectionate attention to child-patients. Although in some situations and particularly with school-age children such volunteers may do good, the concept is generally mistaken as a provision for the under-fours. In the experience of some hospitals which employ the system, volunteers can usually give no more than a few hours each week to the job, which can mean that the child gets his TLC ('tender loving care') from two or three volunteers in a day and perhaps from ten or twenty in a week.

For the under-four this is grossly unsatisfactory, although this may be concealed by his 'settledness' and the fact that no one has real contact with him. Furthermore, such provisions for young children—which in a large hospital can be most elaborately organized with rota charts disposing of several hundred well-meaning people—are reactionary in their influence on policy if, as sometimes happens, they are associated with restricted visiting for

81

parents. In a known instance the effect is that volunteers have more access to young children than do their own parents. And of course the system diverts energy and concern from the vital need to allow adequate access by the mother or to reorganize the nursing system on the 'case-assignment' method. Where play activities are required it is much better that they be provided by full-time paid employees whose work and relationships will have some continuity.

This does not mean that volunteers cannot be of positive value, particularly with older children. But it does mean that their organization is only justified if all other methods of giving basic care through mother and paid staff have already been exploited to the full. The procedure in some hospitals abroad, where the nurse who notices a crying or depressed child marks 'TLC' on his card and leaves it to a series of volunteers to give the 'tender loving care' thus prescribed, illustrates how misconception about the nature of the child's need for love can result in an extreme of absurdity—and how elaborate provision for giving frag-ments of TLC can obscure the essential and urgent problem.

Play

There has been a surge of interest in providing 'play specialists/therapists/ladies' for children in hospital, and insofar as this expresses concern to improve the quality of life for child patients it is to be welcomed. There is no doubt that for older children play can provide interest and fill hours that otherwise might be wearisome. They have the maturity to understand why they are in hospital, to tolerate hours of absence from their parents as they do while at school, and to know precisely when their parents will next visit. Therefore they can fit play into their day and make good use of it while they await confidently for their eventual return home.

But the value of ward play as an activity for the younger patients, for instance for the unaccompanied under-3s, is infinitely less. Some advocates of play tend to imply that as an activity it has comparable importance for children right down to the first months of life, when we are told that babies need the stimulation of bright objects and things to finger. The generalization about the value of play over-looks the simple fact that the primary need of the infant and very young child is not play *per se* but interaction with a warm and responsive mothering person.

This is at best the mother, though in her unavoidable absence a ward foster mother who is wholly available to relate to the child can bring many benefits (127). Whoever looks with knowledge of child development at a very young patient with a play person will be aware that it is not the activity which holds the child but the relationship with the person—and that it is then loss of the person and not loss of the play thing which is distressing. Play persons can rarely stay long enough with any one child to meet the emotional needs of the very young.

Play provisions which do not clearly recognize the special needs of the under-3s may, because of the air of activity they bring to the ward, divert attention from the primary importance of bringing mothers into hospital to help care for their children.

THE TRAINING OF DOCTORS AND NURSES

The training of doctors in this country contains little to help them understand the emotional needs of young children or to detect the subtle ways in which distress or significant psychological disturbance can be shown. The new curriculum for nurses' training has introduced some lectures on the psychology of children, but must still be regarded as inadequate (23, 30, 41).

Isolated experiments in amelioration are made by individuals and groups with unusual intuition, with the limitation that this must have, but not until systematic knowledge is built into trainings can any widespread advance be made. If doctors and nurses are to be more effective in looking after the mental health of young patients their training must include the psychological development of children, coupled with adequate practical experience of normal healthy young children—not only during training but at regular refresher intervals thereafter to ensure that their norms of behaviour remain real. Norms are readily distorted if only sick and separated children are seen.

Training in the dynamics of child behaviour and development would not only add a new and necessary dimension to the work of the medical and nursing professions. It would also enable more doctors and nurses to understand that psychiatrists and others in allied professions carry knowledge and skills as specialized as those in physical medicine and as worthy of respect. It is still too common for paediatricians and physicians to dismiss summarily the judgements of psychiatrists on mental health matters in which they themselves have no training—yet they would be rightly indignant if a worker in the mental health field were to step out of his speciality to make public rejection of a paediatric diagnosis.

The integration of mental health concepts into medical and nursing training will not make doctors and nurses into mental health specialists, but as understanding grows of the essential links between the physical and the emotional it will be realized that there is need for close collaboration with psychiatrists, psycho-analysts, psychologists, and sociologists from whose disciplines these mental health concepts derive (26, 51).

Conclusions

For the convenience of the reader a point-by-point summary of the foregoing matter precedes the presentation of the Conclusions.

THE YOUNG CHILD IN HOSPITAL

In recent years there has been a marked trend towards 'humanizing' the care of young children in hospital. Amenities are being improved—there is increased visiting, provision of playrooms and teachers, and general brightening of surroundings. These innovations are welcome, but it is clear that they are rarely introduced as part of a coherent approach to meeting the child's emotional needs. And because they are commonly *ad hoc* changes and not part of a general application of a basic principle, it is not uncommon to find that the procedures to which a child is subjected are inconsistent with each other and even mutually contradictory in their influence. Thus there may be daily visiting—but no visiting at all for the first two days, 'to give the child time to settle down'; or there may be daily visiting yet the child be abruptly removed from the mother in the admission room; the mother may be allowed to visit before an operation but not be allowed into the induction room to support him into unconsciousness; care may be loving but be applied by so many nurses that the child is not 'mothered'.

The motivation to 'humanize' has many sound procedures to its credit, but unless it is linked to a basic concept of the child's needs which can be applied to all aspects of his experience in hospital it is unlikely that kind intention will achieve its true end.

The child of under four (an arbitrary line is drawn here) is normally intensely attached to his mother and dependent on her for comfort and security. It is a function of his early environment to keep him physically and emotionally secure, thereby helping him to be a stable and adjusted person in later life.

If he loses the care of his mother by coming into hospital, he becomes insecure and fretful, and the 'settling down' that follows is not to be taken at its face value. There is ample evidence that most young children are anxious and aggressive on return from hospital, and that these adverse features sometimes persist for months or years. Even when not prolonged or permanent they are evidence of a period of great stress and unhappiness in the child and every effort should be made to prevent it.

Systematic studies have shown that although improvement in ward management, including the provision of daily visiting and more play opportunities, lowers the incidence of distress in older children it does little to diminish the distress of children under four years of age. 'No amount of love and understanding will make up for the absence of the mother.'

Going to hospital has two main dangers for the child:

(*a*) *The Traumatic*, in which the shock of losing the mother and the other stresses to which he is subjected, which may be cumulative, is greater than his mental structure can master, and a temporary or permanent degree of disequilibrium may result. To the Traumatic the passage of time can add:

(*b*) *The Deprivational*, in which lengthy deprivation of mothering by one person may result in lasting impoverishment of the personality.

Aspects of the foregoing are illustrated by summary accounts of three child patients observed by the author:

(*a*) *A Short Stay in Hospital* describes the behaviour of a child of two during and after eight days in hospital.

(*b*) *A 'Settled' Child* follows into the home a child of three who had been judged to be happily 'settled' during five weeks in hospital.

(*c*) *A Long Stay in Hospital* follows a child through the phases of Protest, Despair, and Denial during eighteen months in hospital begun at the age of two; and describes serious maladaptation persisting a year after return home.

SOME IMPLICATIONS FOR HOSPITAL PRACTICE

ADMISSION OF MOTHER AND CHILD

FAMILIES in less developed cultures and in the most sophisticated and wealthy sections of industrialized societies remain in close contact with their sick, especially with their sick children. But the hospitals on which the greater part of the world's population is dependent restrict contact between parents and their sick children.

The practicability of admitting mothers and children has been demonstrated for many years in isolated units, invariably as an expression of an unusually gifted person or group of people, but there has been much resistance to the idea.

Experience shows that most mothers given the opportunity are eager to come into hospital with their young

children, and with the help of father, relatives, and neighbours will find ways of doing so without imposing undue
hardship on other children in the family. In one ward the
majority of mothers admitted have more than one child,
and various expedients are used to maintain contact
between mothers and children left at home. Most often the
patient is the youngest child in the family, but where there
is a younger child who may be adversely affected by the
absence of the mother special arrangements might have to
be made to ensure adequate contact—for example by
giving him a cot in an adjacent room in the hospital, or
having him in a play group attached to the ward.

The objections are made that resident mothers would
obstruct the work of wards by their presence and by
unreliable behaviour, and that children are more difficult
to manage in the presence of mothers. However, it has
been demonstrated that, if brought into hospital with her
young child and given a proper role in relation to his care,
the ordinary mother will show herself to be as competent
and courageous as she usually is when nursing a sick child
at home under the guidance of the family doctor. Undoubtedly a child is less easy to manage in the presence of
his mother, but ways should be found of accepting this. It
is better for him to protest in her presence than to be
submissive in her absence.

The mother, by her presence and by making explanations to the child, can prevent anxieties and misconceptions
becoming cumulatively overwhelming.

In a good mothers-in unit the mother is not a rival to
the nurse. The nurse's role is enriched, not least by the
understanding she gains of the mother-child relationship
but also by the support she can give to the mother in
difficult situations.

Attention is drawn to two relevant publications:

Young Children in Hospital

(a) *Film: Going to Hospital with Mother*, in which a mother is admitted to hospital with her child of 20 months, and there attends to her simple care. The child remains secure in her mother's presence, and neither in hospital nor afterwards does she show any of the fretfulness or other forms of disturbed behaviour commonly seen in young children who go to hospital unaccompanied.

(b) *Paper: 'A Mother's Observations on the Tonsillectomy of Her Four-Year-Old Daughter'*, in which a mother who was admitted to hospital with her child gives a detailed account of the child's behaviour before, during, and after her stay in hospital.

Unless the social role of mothers is understood and valued, having mothers in will be unsatisfactory.

The need for training is stressed, to ensure that the establishment and survival of units for mothers and children does not depend on outstanding personalities but on knowledge.

VISITING AND SYSTEMS OF NURSING

Visiting   (a) *Some General Considerations*

In general there should be no restriction on visiting times, and parents should be left to decide for themselves how much they will visit—with help when necessary to resolve their anxieties about it.

During visits the parents should be free, subject to overriding medical considerations, to do much of the ordinary care.

If visiting is restricted it should be understood that the child's crying is a normal and inevitable reaction, and the nurse should show sympathetic understanding and try to comfort.

To maintain links with home between visits the child should have his favourite 'cuddly' or toy, which should on no account be taken from him. An object which the child knows the mother values and will return for can also be left, such as a glove or purse. Postcards and letters that nurse will read for him should be encouraged. At the end of visits the child, if old enough, should be told truthfully by his parents that they are going, and a familiar nurse should stand by to comfort him.

It is mistaken to regard daily visiting as a panacea and the goal of reform. Welcome advance though the provision is, such research as has been done shows clearly that the daily visit does not provide adequate contact between the young child and his mother and remains associated with much stress.

Visiting (b) *In Fever Hospitals*

Many fever (isolation) hospitals allow no visiting, generally on grounds that infection may be conveyed into the community. The fact that some fever hospitals do permit visiting, subject to certain precautions affecting clothing and contact, suggests that not all of the objections are reasonable.

One fever hospital which allows daily visiting reports that there is no evidence that this has been responsible for the transmission of infection to the community. It has led to improved morale of all fever patients, both adults and children, and to improvement in the public relations of the hospital.

Systems of Nursing

'Work-assignment' nursing, which involves most nurses on the ward in the care of each child, may deal efficiently with the physical needs of the young patient but does not satisfy his need for attachment and security.

'Team or group assignment', in which a small team of nurses care for a small group of patients is a great advance on 'work assignment' but is still not the optimum provision.

'Case-assignment' nursing gives each nurse a small family group of mixed ages. She feeds, toilets, and generally attends to all aspects of the body care of each of her patients. This gives the young child opportunity for individual attachment and for the expression of the normal range of feeling and behaviour, and the security of a stable relationship.

The nursing should be so organized that on off-times and off-days only one or two known nurses act as relief.

If the nurse is a student she should not move to another ward until her 'family' has been discharged.

If the children are long-stay, the nurse should be permanent and not a student.

Since children cared for by case assignment will become attached to their nurse and show the normal variations of behaviour of the family child, it will be necessary to give the nurse opportunities for training and for advice on the behaviour of her patients, and, subject to overriding medical considerations, to allow her considerable discretion in the management of her own 'family'.

THE SPECIAL PROBLEM OF THE LONG-STAY WARD

Similar considerations apply to long-stay as to short-stay children—the need for the mother's presence and for 'case-assignment nursing'—but the problem is more serious because length of stay and distance from home would generally make it impossible for a mother to come into residence or to visit adequately.

Visiting should be unrestricted.

Nursing should be by permanent nurses on 'case assignment' or, much preferable where practicable, by lay foster-mothers providing maternal-type care under the control of a lay head trained in child development.

The latter notion conceives of wards being structured as children's homes with medical and technical nursing attention available, but with all 'non-medical' care given by foster-mothers. This would raise the standard of 'substitute mothering' to the level now being achieved in institutions for healthy children.

The occupation offered to young children confined to their cots for long periods should include ample opportunity for aggressive and noisy play—e.g. with hammer-pegs, drums, etc.—and for messy play with sand, water, and finger-paints.

PREPARATION OF THE YOUNG CHILD FOR HOSPITAL

The younger the child the more difficult it is to do any worthwhile preparation. It is doubtful if under-threes can be helped in this way.

Preparation will be more effective if done by the parents and supported in the event by frequent visiting.

Preparation should be simple and truthful, but not more than the child can assimilate.

The aim should be to give an honest picture of the strange environment into which he has to go, and to give reassurance that he will return.

If there is to be an operation, the pain should be mentioned—coupled with assurance that it will get better.

He should not be told too far ahead about going to hospital, perhaps beginning a week in advance with a first intimation and supplementing at the pace set by his questions. But if he learns by chance some weeks ahead, for instance by overhearing parents or doctors talk about it, it is best to answer his questions as from then.

In the two-and-a-half- to three-year-old age group little preparation can be done, but games of going away and coming back may help a little.

Still younger children cannot be prepared in any way. This confirms the absolute necessity for basing their care on the presence and participation of the mother.

It is also impossible to prepare for emergency admissions.

If a child has a favourite toy or a 'thing' which he holds or sucks when frightened, tired, or unwell, it should always be available to him in hospital. Even if his comforter is a 'dummy' ('pacifier' in America) he should not be deprived of it.

Parents can be helped to prepare their children through the right kind of leaflet, i.e. one that is realistic about the problem without detailing incidental treatments and does not omit to deal with hurt, tears, and post-separation disturbances in behaviour. The ability of parents to deal with the painful task of preparation would be much improved if they could meet a suitable staff member a week or two before admission to discuss the matter.

A NOTE ON THE FEELINGS OF PARENTS

Parents also need consideration if their young child goes to hospital. Although they are grateful for the skill and attention that are available there, they are justifiably apprehensive about the unhappiness that separation from them will inevitably mean for their child.

If they have to give the child over entirely to the hospital, and are not allowed to visit freely or help in his care, their self-esteem—especially that of the mother—may be seriously undermined. The resultant sense of inadequacy may be intensified if the child is difficult to manage on return home. Recalling that he was docile and 'well-behaved' with the nurses, the mother may feel disappointed and incompetent. This may affect her ability to be tolerant and patient with the disturbances in his behaviour.

The mother who is allowed to visit freely and to do things for her child will remain realistic in her view of him—and her self-esteem will be sustained. Her anxieties will be appropriate to the illness. She will be the more competent to take over his care on return home and, incidentally, since their close relationship was maintained the transition from hospital to home will be greatly eased.

THE REASSESSMENT OF HOSPITAL PROCEDURES

To ensure that the benefits of good provisions are not vitiated by others that are unnecessarily distressing, routines and procedures should be constantly scrutinized to evaluate their necessity.

The persistence of out-dated routines and procedures can cause kindly staff to be unwittingly inconsiderate, and it requires conscious effort to stand aside from established practice in order to assess its significance.

Examples are given of the way in which routines can override consideration for child and parent, and of how this might be avoided.

The question is raised whether masks, which can be very frightening to young children, need be worn as often as they are.

To minimize anxiety the young child should have a nurse whom he knows to be his 'special' nurse. She should accompany him and his mother through all reception procedures, and be present at all treatments and investigations whether mother is able to stay or not. Even apparently minor matters need consideration. For instance, the young patient should not be moved from one ward to another, or from ward to cubicle, unless accompanied by his mother and 'special' nurse. He can become very afraid that his mother will not find him again if he is moved from the place where she last saw him.

Two provisions which are generally misconceived although well-intentioned are:

(a) That all members of professional staff should pick up a child on each transit through the ward.

(b) That 'volunteers' should be organized to give occupation and affectionate attention to young patients.

Both of these give fragmented attention which is unhelpful and confusing to the child; and the latter in particular, with its large investment in organization and good intention, may seriously delay recognition of the hospital's responsibility to provide security and love through the mother and/or permanent staff.

THE TRAINING OF DOCTORS AND NURSES

There is little in the present training of doctors and nurses to help them understand the emotional needs of young children or to detect the subtle ways in which distress or significant psychological disturbance can be shown. Trainings should be expanded to include the dynamics of child behaviour and development, coupled with adequate experience of normal healthy children to ensure that norms are not distorted.

Such training will not make doctors and nurses into

mental health specialists, but in addition to adding a new and necessary dimension to their work it will bring greater recognition that those who work in psychiatry and allied professions carry knowledge and skills as specialized as those in medicine. As understanding grows of the link between the physical and the mental it will be found that there is much scope for productive collaboration between the paediatric and the psychiatric.

CONCLUSIONS

The purpose of this short book has been to outline a principle of mental health and to indicate some of the implications for the kind of 'non-medical and non-nursing' care necessary to protect the social and emotional development of young children in hospital. Little attempt has been made to go into detail, though considerations of what is practical have been kept in mind.

The primary need of young children is for a 'warm, intimate and continuous relationship to the mother, or to a mother-substitute, in which they both find satisfaction and enjoyment'. It has been argued that admitting the mother with the child, or permitting unrestricted visiting by the mother, best meet this need; and that the 'case-assignment' system of nursing, in short-term wards in particular, and the re-structuring of long-stay wards as children's homes with lay foster-mothers, would be the next best provision in the unavoidable absence of the mother.

An important function of the mother or mother substitute in the hospital situation is, by her presence and explanations, to help the child keep anxiety in check and within the limits of tolerance. Anxieties can be cumulative in their effect, and it is most important that the positive influence of mother or mother substitute should be supported by procedures within the hospital that are reassessed to ensure that they cause the minimum of stress to the child.

An inevitable consequence of innovations in the directions recommended would be that young patients would show a more normal range of emotions and behaviour. This the nurse will be able to deal with only if, subject to overriding medical considerations, she is given more latitude with her charges. An implication is that the training of doctors and nurses should be extended to include a dynamic view of the emotional development of children, coupled with practical experience of normal healthy children. Every children's ward should have available to it the services of a senior staff member with appropriate qualifications in child development, to give seminars on general and particular aspects of child behaviour and to be available to advise on individual children.

Postscript 1970

In 1959 the Committee[1] appointed by the Ministry of Health[2] published its long-awaited Report, *The Welfare of Children in Hospital* (102). During a period of two years, evidence had been taken from the professions associated with hospitals—nursing, medicine, psychiatry, social work, administration. The 'Platt Report',[3] so named after the distinguished surgeon who headed the inquiry, made a detailed series of recommendations about the 'non-medical' aspects of the care of child patients from birth to sixteen years.

The three recommendations that drew most attention were:

(*a*) that visiting to all children should be unrestricted; this was later defined by the Minister of Health to mean that parents should be allowed to visit at any time during which children could reasonably be expected to be awake;

[1] The Committee of 12 comprised: 2 paediatricians, 1 physician, 2 surgeons, 1 psychiatrist, 2 nurses, 2 hospital administrators, 1 hospital headmistress, 1 lay member (woman).

[2] In 1969 the Ministry of Health was replaced by the Department of Health and Social Security, and the functions of the Minister of Health were taken over by the Secretary of State for Health and Social Security.

[3] Unless otherwise specified, reference throughout is to the Platt Report of 1959. Sir Harry Platt was also Chairman of a Committee investigating nurse training whose report published in 1964 (129) is also known as the 'Platt Report'.

(b) that provision should be made to enable mothers of children under five years of age to stay with them in hospital, in order to help in their care and prevent the distress and risks to mental health associated with separation;

(c) that the training of medical and nursing students should be improved to give them greater understanding of the emotional needs of children.

The Platt Report got a very warm welcome from both the professional and the lay press. It was clear that the recommendations touched upon something that everyone knew to be good and true in human relations. Parents who wished to stay close to a young child in hospital now had the support both of expert opinion and of government policy, and could with propriety no longer be treated as fussy and over-concerned.

But humane and reasonable though the recommendations of the Report are, it was not to be expected that they would be speedily implemented in all children's wards. In established institutions, traditional beliefs and practices tend to persist long after their inappropriateness has been demonstrated. This is perhaps especially true of hospitals. Methods of ward management that have proved efficient and convenient in the treatment of illness are not readily modified to suit considerations of mental health, especially if these considerations are insufficiently understood. Furthermore, doctors and nurses in hospitals have for so long had the role of doing things *for* people that the concept of doing things *with* people—e.g. with parents—is one that takes root very slowly. A Report, however much applauded, cannot change overnight the practices and attitudes of generations.

The recommendations of the Platt Report were adopted

as official Ministry of Health policy, but the policy could not be enforced—for the reason that it is not possible to legislate on matters of professional judgement. Therefore, although in statements in the House of Commons and in circulars to all hospitals the Minister of Health asked that the recommendations be implemented, he refrained from issuing directives. It was left to the professions to improve their children's ward practice at the pace at which the importance of the recommendations was understood—with the encouragement of regular inquiries from the Minister about progress, and the occasional issue of statistics allowing comparisons to be made.

By the time the Report was published in 1959, a number of senior hospital paediatricians, influenced by the changing climate of thought, had already gone a long way in humanizing their ward procedures; in addition, a method of bringing hospital care into the home, as a way of preventing or minimizing hospitalization, had begun and continues to function successfully (10, 36, 37, 59, 82, 89, 93, 117, 118, 132). But the Platt Report gave a fresh impetus to the trend towards change. Quite junior people, who until then had had little opportunity to try out their progressive ideas, could now use the authority of the Report to get the support of their superiors.

The next few years saw a substantial easing of visiting restrictions and positive moves to involve parents in tending child patients. Many wards now have some provision for the accommodation of mothers, and there are a number of prototypes of the adequate children's ward—where visiting is unrestricted and where mothers of children under five are encouraged to stay. There is no doubt that these wards are very successful. We see in them a fresh balance of relationships in which doctors, nurses, orderlies, and mothers combine to provide the best possible care. The mother is not there on sufferance or as a concession to sentiment, but has a genuine role in the care of her child. The child does not become depressed and withdrawn, as unaccompanied children commonly do. Because of the presence of the mother he retains the spontaneity and free expression of feeling of the young child in the security of his own home (120). [One of these wards, whose good practice was established well ahead of the Report, is the subject of a film (117, 118, 137).]

However, this has not been a uniform development throughout the country. Instances where ward practice has been improved, and in particular where prototypes of the good mother–child unit have appeared, have been sporadic and dependent more upon concern to prevent manifest distress than upon acceptance of mental health considerations.[1] The advent of a good mother–child unit has usually turned upon there being a chance constellation of like-minded people or upon a highly motivated paediatrician being able to inspire his juniors to face the problems and discover the benefits of change. As long as these prototypes depend upon the humanity of the paediatrician and nurse in charge there is no guarantee of their survival, or of their good example being followed. This can only be assured when the training of medical and nursing students gives adequate understanding of the emotional needs of children, as the Platt Report recommends.

THE PRESSURE OF AN INFORMED PUBLIC OPINION

There was a distinct danger that, a major but uneven step forward having been taken, inertia would re-establish

[1] A distinguished paediatrician whose ward practice is second to none has written: "Our primary concern is to prevent the unhappiness that is caused to young patients by separation from the mother. The possibility of after-effects or lasting effects from separation has always been a secondary consideration. . . ." (118).

itself and that sections of the country would continue to be served by wards whose practice had changed little or not at all. The question then was to what extent general improvement could be obtained without waiting long years until better trainings had been devised and their influence felt. Until 1959, when the Platt Report was published, the Tavistock had scrupulously confined its teaching and propaganda on the problem to the hospital professions in order to give them opportunity to come to terms with the findings of research, and in particular with the impact of the films *A Two-Year-Old Goes to Hospital* and *Going to Hospital With Mother* (6, 10). But when the Platt Report made the issue a public one, it was decided that the time had come to help to create an informed public opinion that would press and persuade hospitals everywhere in the country to implement the Report, and in particular to show that parents and staff had complementary roles in securing the well-being of the young patient.

The two films were released for public discussion under knowledgeable leadership, and in 1961 they were shown on television discussion programmes in which paediatricians, nurses, and parents took part. Simultaneously a series of articles contributed by the author to a quality newspaper urged community pressure to hasten the implementation of the Platt Report (102). These presentations produced a great number of letters about good and bad experiences of children's wards, later published in book form (120), and also led to the founding of the National Association for the Welfare of Children in Hospital (N.A.W.C.H.)[1] by a group of young parents who had the intelligence and education both to understand

[1] Originally called Mother Care for Children in Hospital. Address: National Association for the Welfare of Children in Hospital, 74 Dennison House, Vauxhall Bridge Road, London, SW1 (01-834-1124).

the issues and not to be intimidated by medical authority.

Among the original members of N.A.W.C.H. were parents whose children had had bad hospital experiences, and understandably they felt like attacking the hospitals that were resistant to change. But this would have hardened resistances and alienated the sympathies even of progressive doctors and nurses. It was found possible to work in a constructive and reconciling way that acknowledged that parents and hospital staffs have a common concern to do what is best for child patients even though, for historical reasons, there remain differences of view as to what is necessary.

N.A.W.C.H. is now a thriving national movement with more than 50 groups and 4,000 members throughout Britain. These organize public meetings, and infiltrate the topic of children in hospital into the syllabuses of other organizations. With the Platt Report as their blueprint, N.A.W.C.H. groups visit their local hospitals to discuss how far the recommendations have been implemented and what intentions there are of doing so. Since the Minister of Health did not seek to compel implementation, but left it to the professions to move towards change at their own pace, this lobbying by local groups is of enormous importance.

Generally the exchanges between N.A.W.C.H. and hospital authorities are cordial and have done much to dispel mutual misconceptions in the course of understanding each other's problems. This lay-initiated movement has excellent standing in the community, and a consistently good national press. The membership includes a growing number of paediatricians, doctors, nurses, hospital administrators, social workers, and hospital play leaders, many of whom are actively involved in the work of the Association. They serve as consultants, share platforms with parents at public meetings, and thus indirectly help their colleagues towards more realistic and sympathetic appreciation of ordinary parents.

The movement has other activities. Whenever official statistics are issued on visiting and other facilities in children's wards, N.A.W.C.H. produces the figures of its latest relevant survey for comparison, and when necessary points to discrepancies between official statement and actual practice. N.A.W.C.H. also keeps check on the shifts and changes in children's wards throughout the country, and is able to advise and help parents to get their children into the kind of ward that best suits them; and although N.A.W.C.H. policy is mainly one of gentle and reasonable persuasion it will, when urgent need arises and the well-being of a child is at risk, support parents by intervening with the administration to overcome the prohibitions of a restrictive ward. N.A.W.C.H. groups run baby-sitter and transport services for parents, and in several places they have raised money for specially built mother–child accommodation; they have also provided both voluntary and salaried play leaders.

In consultation with doctors, nurses, and administrators, N.A.W.C.H. produced a most successful Hospital Admission leaflet which is sold to hospitals for distribution to parents (109). Within two years of publication in October 1967, 84,000 leaflets had been sold.

A handful of consultant paediatricians are tireless in their practical support of N.A.W.C.H., ready not only to advise but also to take effective action when their special knowledge and authority can promote a venture or give weight to an expression of concern at the hurtful consequences of restrictive practices. An instance of this occurred in 1965, when two consultant paediatricians responded to the grief of an unmarried mother over the death of her three-year-old child by contributing to *The Lancet* a profound comment on the tragic consequences of the mother having been prevented from visiting the child in hospital (92).

Reliable information is hard to obtain but, according to N.A.W.C.H., in 1970 perhaps 160 (20 per cent) of the 800 hospitals that admit children have 'some' accommodation for mothers. About 64 (8 per cent) are said to offer accommodation routinely, and about 96 (12 per cent) will provide a bed for a mother in certain circumstances.[1]

The few wards with a positive policy of involving parents attract a high rate of usage, and the practice of mothers accompanying their young children into hospital becomes an accepted part of the local culture. (At Amersham General Hospital and in the paediatric wards at Stoke Mandeville Hospital, for instance, the majority of children under five are now accompanied by their mothers —or fathers! Since these local hospitals also have totally unrestricted visiting, parents can use the facilities in whatever ways suit their individual circumstances. A high level of parent–child contact is thus achieved.)

In many of the other hospital wards with 'some' accommodation, this is used sparingly for mothers deemed by the physician to' be 'suitable', or for the strong-minded mother who presses her wish to stay with her child. But in the great majority of children's wards there is still no provision for the accommodation of mothers. However, the point has been reached where, provided it is not an emergency admission, any mother who wishes to stay with her young child in hospital can usually be found a place quite quickly through the co-operation of the more enlightened paediatricians—

---

[1] In addition, about 200 hospitals say they will accommodate mothers of 'seriously ill' children, and about 160 will admit breast-feeding mothers.

provided she is willing to travel to another part of the country if necessary. Some mothers do this.

Although a certain amount of improvement has come about in the last decade, there remain areas of resistance and some indication of retrogression. A 1969 survey by N.A.W.C.H. showed that only 57 per cent of children's hospitals in the South West Metropolitan Region allowed unrestricted visiting, defined for the survey at a modest 45 hours per week. This sampling in a prosperous area is a corrective to the 'national average' of 85 per cent claimed by the Department of Health. (The Department's statement was based on figures got at hospital administration level, but N.A.W.C.H.'s surveys have repeatedly shown that these are usually inaccurate when compared with figures got at ward level.)

Of the 65 hospitals surveyed, '16 had some mothers' beds, 10 would find one in an emergency, and 3 had a bed for the mother only if the child was a private patient and the mother could pay; in the remaining 36 hospitals no arrangements could be made for the mother to stay' (110).

In 1969 much less visiting was being allowed in tonsils wards than two years earlier, and of 24 hospitals investigated in various parts of the country only 8 could provide a bed for the mother of a child undergoing tonsillectomy. In 4 of these hospitals accommodation was for private patients only at £8 a night.

These statistics can be understood mainly in terms of continuing lack of understanding of the importance of preserving the bond between the young child and his mother. Ten years after the Platt Report N.A.W.C.H. understandably found the situation 'extremely disappointing' (110).

This suggests that there is a limit to what can be

achieved by persuasion and appeal to the humanity of the hospital professions. It may be that a plateau has been reached, and that further progress will not be made until greater understanding of the psychological development and emotional needs of children is built into medical and nursing training—in line with an urgent recommendation of the Platt Report, 1959.

It is not only that improvements in practice are uneven as between hospitals and as between different parts of the country, but that even within the more humane wards incompatible practices may be found. In a ward that actively encourages mothers to stay, the care of un-accompanied young children may be no better than elsewhere. For lack of conviction about the importance of mothering *per se*, the unaccompanied child may still be looked after in traditional ways that fragment his care among shifts and changes of nurses, instead of by patient assignment, which is the only way to meet the child's need of a substitute mother.

Consistency in meeting the emotional needs of young patients requires knowledge, insight, and understanding. There must be an integrating principle of care. It is not enough that the physician is a kindly father-figure and that the ward sister loves children. Kind intention can achieve much, but can be blind to the subtler manifestations of need, and is of itself no substitute for the precise knowledge of psychological development that comes only through relevant training.

Since so much depends upon trainings that are either nonexistent or still rudimentary in form, it will clearly be many years before paediatric care conforms to modern knowledge of child development. But at the highest levels of administration there appears to be optimism that the major objectives will be attained in due course. It has been accepted by the Department of Health that no charge need or should be made for the accommodation of mothers when they stay with their children in hospital, that the presence of the mother is not a luxury but an essential part of enlightened hospital care. At that level it is well understood that the hospital staff have as their main task to deal with the child's illness, while the mother by her presence keeps the child secure and so helps safeguard his later mental health.

Furthermore, in the planning of new hospitals the Government is taking a positive long-term view. It is laid down as a requirement that for every twenty beds serving children from birth to sixteen years there shall be at least four rooms suitable for the accommodation together of mothers and young children (103, 104). The implication is that in due course it will be routine practice to admit mothers and young children together, and that the hospital professions and parents alike will by then understand the necessity for doing so.

Another important publication with an eye to the future is the Nuffield Foundation's *Children in Hospital: Studies in Planning* (112). This presents the findings of a research unit that included paediatricians, nurses, sociologists, architects, and epidemiologists, and describes and illustrates with detailed drawings the implications of the Platt Report for hospital design. Under this plan new children's wards would be designed on a flexible basis with divans for mothers recessed into the walls so that they do not encumber the rooms. An incidental advantage would be that during the phase of transition any paediatrician who was not 'with it' could continue with out-of-date practice, but that the next generation of paediatricians and nurses would inherit structures fully suited to the routine admission of mothers and children.

Young Children in Hospital

The Platt Report was an historic and humane document that precipitated many advances in the care of hospitalized children. But in some respects the Report did not adequately reflect the expert psychological knowledge that was made available to the Committee.

It is a psychological truism that if a small child loses the care of his mother he has urgent need of a stable relationship with a warm and responsive mother-figure if his emotional needs are to be met (1). But the Platt Committee apparently did not fully appreciate the implications of this principle of mental health, and their recommendations for practice are therefore inadequate. Thus, although the Report urges the desirability of mothers accompanying their small children into hospital, the recommendation is diminished by the qualification 'for the first few days'. This appears to be on the assumption that after a few days the small patient will be so much at ease in the ward that he will not mind his mother leaving.

The assumption ignores the nature of small children, especially when ill, which is such that *whenever* the mother leaves a separation begins to which the dependent young child will respond with acute distress. It also overlooks the fact that when the mother is not there the child will rarely if ever find a substitute mother among the shifts and changes of ward staff.

This lack of adequate conviction about the importance of ongoing warm and responsive mothering, and the need to provide it in the absence of the mother, is still more serious in relation to the care of long-stay patients. Although the Report recognizes that mothers are usually unable to maintain close contact with their children in long-stay wards, there is no mention of the serious problem of how the young patient's need of mothering is to be met. Yet if mothering is important for the short-stay child, how much more important must it be for the small child who is in the hospital for months or years?

The problem is of such a different order of severity from that of the short-stay ward that it was quite inadequate for the Report to say, almost *en passant*, that 'most of our recommendations apply equally to long-stay hospitals' (102, para. 117). For the long-stay young patient there is a high probability of severe emotional deprivation because of the prolonged separation and the lack of stable mothering care. But there is little in the Platt Report to convey that this is a grave situation that threatens the mental health of long-stay young patients (102, para. 117, a-f).

It is sometimes said that nowadays fewer young children are in hospital for lengthy periods, that many are sent home between brief periods of treatment. This is true; but if a child is a number of times in and out of hospital the *total* length of stay may be long. Furthermore, he will have repeated separations from the mother to endure, each aggravating the experience of the previous ones. For the child who is in and out of hospital it is just as important as for the truly long-stay child that his emotional needs are provided for.

Not so many years ago it was widely held that small children could be happy in short-stay wards when separated from the mother and with restricted visiting. That myth is now exploded. But another myth remains, which is that all is well in long-stay wards.

It is perhaps not surprising that the myth lingers, in neglect of what is known of child development and the responses of young children to separation and deprivation of mothering care. Young patients in long-stay wards are

111

often bright and friendly, or at least quiet and uncomplaining, and the visitor is readily disarmed by this and by the atmosphere of kindliness and busyness with education and nursery-school play. Perhaps it was the reassurance of this superficially charming picture that caused the Platt Committee to put aside expert evidence about the psychological damage that underlies the blandness and easy friendliness so often found in long-stay young patients. As has been described earlier in this book (pages 11-18), such children have passed through the stages of Protest and Despair and their adapted and uncomplaining behaviour has been achieved at the heavy cost of Denial (now called Detachment).

The National Association for the Welfare of Children in Hospital is now pressing for operational research to be done in long-stay wards (121). Some of the proposals that such an operational project might investigate are outlined on pages 63-68 of this book. Notice should also be taken of recent experience in the United States of the value of salaried foster-grandparents in children's wards (88, 134).

The basic needs of all small children, healthy or sick, are the same. Current studies by the author and his wife on the influence of certain variables on the responses of healthy young children to separation from the mother, especially the presence or absence of stable and responsive substitute mothering, are therefore relevant to the care of hospitalized children.

In one part of these studies close observation of *John*, a child of seventeen months admitted to a residential nursery, showed how the fragmented care of changing nurses failed to meet his need of mothering, and provoked extreme separation responses of a classical kind. This is on film (70, 124, 127). An implication for hospital care is that the common practice of having young patients handled by a number of nurses must frustrate the need for a stable mother-figure and contribute greatly to the distress of the young patient who is not accompanied by his mother (113).

Furthermore, in the background to *John* are a number of small children who have been in the institution for a long time. Their superficially bright and diverting behaviour is shown to be aggressive, self-centred, ruthless, promiscuous. They have no close relationships and are not sad when nurses leave. There is a parallel between the emotionally impoverished state of these healthy deprived children and the condition of long-stay young patients in hospital wards.

The young child who is away from his family, whether healthy or in hospital, must be given *warm* and responsive substitute mothering if his mental health is to be safeguarded.

THE HOSPITAL PROFESSIONS AND THE PLATT REPORT

In accepting the Platt Report in 1959, the Minister of Health did not seek to enforce the recommendations but tacitly put the onus upon the hospital professions to bring about better practice on the basis of improved trainings for medical and nursing students. What, then, have the medical and nursing professions done about this in the ten years that have elapsed? And what of the lay committees that in theory govern our hospitals and that, as representatives of the community, might be expected to play an important part in obtaining implementation of the Platt Report?

Young Children in Hospital

(a) The Doctors
The Platt Report of 1959 said:

'. . . the training of medical and nursing students takes too little account of the child's emotional and mental needs (para. 11) . . . all who have to look after sick children should learn not only how to deal with the child's ailment but also how to meet his emotional and other needs (para. 137).

But ten years later there is little improvement in the teaching of medical students, in whose syllabuses paediatrics is often a second-class subject. A 1966 survey of 26 undergraduate medical schools showed that half had a professor of paediatrics and half did not, 40 per cent of the students were taught in departments without university status, and the time spent on paediatric firms varied from 8 to 12 weeks (100 hours to 314). Furthermore:

'In medical schools without university departments it is usually chance alone which decides whether the paediatrics teacher is a member of the academic board of the school. . . . There are no standards for paediatric teaching in this country. The importance of paediatrics in the curricula and the facilities for its teaching in many medical schools depend to a great extent on factors other than a reasoned view of what the student requires. It would not be unreasonable to draw the conclusion that in 1966 the condition of at least half the paediatric centres is not up to standard' (81).

Current paediatric teaching deals mainly with the physical aspects; little is taught about the dynamics of child development, the significance of the mother–child relationship, or the psychological meaning to children of

114

illness, pain, and surgical intervention (11, 32, 44, 61, 69, 91, 133). The Royal Commission on Medical Education of 1968 said that 'by and large current teaching in the behavioural sciences to medical students is sketchy' and stressed the need for more systematic teaching (130). This in effect repeated the comment and urgent recommendations made in the Platt Report of ten years earlier.

The poor status of training in child health, and the implications this has for the hopes of further improving the handling of young children in hospitals, is further reflected in the ambiguous standing of the consultant paediatrician. 'There appears to be no approved method by which a young doctor wishing to enter the specialist field of paediatrics can embark on a complete training programme in a university teaching department' (81). He has at present to get relevant experience by applying for jobs here and there, and if he fails to get this or that job he may in due course become a paediatrician with significant gaps in his experience. 'A satisfactory higher diploma has still to be evolved' (80, 85).

The Royal Commission on Medical Education urged that every medical school should have a University Department of Paediatrics headed by a professor, and that teaching should include the growth and development of normal children and an introduction to child psychology (129).

Even if the young doctor overcomes the difficulties created by the lack of a complete training programme at university level and in due course becomes a consultant paediatrician, the probability is that, although an authority on diseases of children, he will have had little or no training in their psychological development—a child specialist who does not have real understanding of children as individuals. The British paediatrician who runs a humane ward does so despite his training. By personal initiative he may seek to fill some of the void by attending informal seminars run by lay child therapists and others, sometimes with difficulty because of age and lengthy habituation to physical paediatrics. Or, like many of the paediatricians in the Health Service, he may soldier on in the conviction that kindness and common sense are better guides than the specialized knowledge of the psychologist or child therapist.

This lack of training in what should be a major component within the speciality of paediatrics, dynamic understanding of the child, could explain the paradox of recent years that some of those resistant to the reforms called for by the Platt Report have been eminent paediatricians; and that, contrary to the hopes of the Platt Committee that they would set a good example to the professions, teaching hospitals have been among the slowest to move.

The memorandum submitted by the British Paediatric Association to the Platt Committee is a lucid and comprehensive exposition of the arrangements and procedures necessary to the humane care and treatment of children in hospital (64). These range from advocacy of home-care schemes as a means of reducing admissions to hospital, unambiguous commitment to unrestricted visiting and the admission of mothers, concern for considerate management of painful treatments, to respect for the individual differences between children as people. There was also a sound proposal, not taken up by the Platt Committee, that '. . . the board of governors or hospital management committee of a general hospital should set up standing sub-committees of lay, paediatric, and nursing members to consider the total well-being of children in their hospital'.

But one major shortcoming of the paediatricians'

memorandum illustrates a limitation of the purely humanitarian approach. Understanding of psychological considerations would have required a section on the kind of nursing care that is necessary for unaccompanied young patients; but this is missing. Although the admission of mothers is advocated, its purpose is imperfectly understood. Concern attaches solely to obtaining the presence of the natural mother, and not to the importance of ensuring continuity of mothering. experience *per se*. Therefore no attention is given to the emotional needs of the young child who is admitted without the mother. The grievous problem of long-stay children is not mentioned.[1]

Another limitation is the implied assumption that concepts of humane care are static and in the realm of sentiment rather than of science, and that they will spread mainly by conversion and contagion. The run of paediatricians are presumed to 'know' what needs to be known, and to take their stand thereon as they might on matters of opinion such as politics and religion. Because it is not understood that human behaviour and relationships are in the area of science, and as such require constant clinical and technical investigation, these matters have little representation on the programmes of paediatric meetings.

A look through recent programmes of the weekend conferences that the British Paediatric Association holds twice a year discovers that the twenty to twenty-five items in each event are concerned almost entirely with

---

[1] The resistance that even progressive paediatricians may have to the findings of psychological research is exampled by question-begging *non sequiturs* that are uncharacteristic of the remainder of the memorandum:

'It is recognised that the admission of a young child to hospital, involving separation from home, may be a misfortune quite apart from the misfortune of the illness itself. Even where a young child is concerned the misfortune is not often serious, especially if the stay in hospital is short. The older child seldom suffers any lasting ill-effects.'

physical disease or gross mental abnormality. The topics of normal emotional development and the meaning of illness and pain to the child are virtually absent.

To revert to the memorandum submitted to the Platt Committee, it is clear that this admirable document reflected the intelligence and compassion of the sub-committee that prepared it, presumably appointed because of their individual concerns, but that it did not represent the consensus of the British Paediatric Association. Otherwise, ten years after Platt, the 300 paediatricians with hospital appointments in the Health Service would be running approximately that number of wards with unrestricted visiting and active policies of including parents in the care of hospitalized children; and the British Paediatric Association would be giving a vigorous lead to the hospital professions in these matters.

That this situation does not exist, and that ten years after Platt it is the lay N.A.W.C.H. movement that struggles to bring about reform, is a sombre comment upon the current status of paediatrics. For lack of appropriate training it will be a long time before a generation of paediatricians appears to whom the safeguarding of emotional well-being can be safely entrusted.

(*b*) *The Nurses*
(i) *The General Nursing Council*. Nurse training throughout England and Wales is based upon a syllabus laid down by the General Nursing Council, a statutory body set up by Act of Parliament in 1919 and required to report annually to the Minister of Health. The General Nursing Council also inspects all nurse training schools and advises on training and examinations (58). Within this integrated system there is therefore much greater opportunity to obtain steady improvement in the psycho-

logical component of training than exists in the complex of highly autonomous medical schools.

In 1959 the Platt Report spoke directly and with special urgency to the nursing profession. After stressing that 'all who have to look after sick children should learn not only how to deal with the child's ailment but also how to meet his emotional and other needs', the Report goes on:

'All this requires special study, and we trust that those responsible for nursing curricula will give all possible priority to the adaptation of nursing courses for the purpose. A few lectures are not enough: experience with normal children in a nursery school . . . would be a great advantage. . . .' (102, para. 139).

In fact, the essential elements of the psychological teaching for which the Platt Report called had already been in the nursing syllabus for the previous seven years but had lain virtually disregarded by the profession. The 1952 syllabus, in which 'Psychology for Nurses' appeared for the first time, contained the following:

'*The Basis of Mental Health.* Security in the mother-child relationship, security in the family situation; love, consistency, discipline and freedom, recognition and praise. *Mother and Child.* Beginnings of capacity to form human relationships, sucking, mothering, weaning, toilet training, effects of separation from the mother, rejection and over-protection' (71).

In 1951 some 42 per cent of British children's wards allowed no visiting, or less than once a week. In one of the provinces as many as 63 per cent did not allow visiting, and in the London area the figure was 36 per cent (84). Tutors and ward sisters were products of the even more restrictive past. Most of them had neither the competence nor the empathy to cope meaningfully with a new syllabus that sought acceptance of the dependence of the young child upon his family.

Had the introduction of 'Psychology for Nurses' into the syllabus in 1952 reflected recognition by the General Nursing Council of a serious and dangerous gap in nurse training, plans would have been laid as a matter of urgency to obtain adequate upgrading within a stated time. There might have been a five- or ten-year plan to establish a body of suitably qualified nurse tutors and 'refreshed' ward sisters. But this did not happen.

As was seen with the paediatricians, psychological knowledge is of a kind that meets with resistance from those whose training is in physical care. Feelings, and the dangers of early separation and maternal deprivation, are less easily understood than the afflictions of the body. Therefore, although nominal acceptance may be given to mental health considerations, lack of conviction stands as an obstacle to effective action. It was presumably for this reason that, although the fundamentals of good psychological development within the mother–child relationship were brought into the 1952 syllabus, the General Nursing Council did not find it necessary to take vigorous action to extend the training of tutors and ward sisters. 'Psychology for Nurses' was left virtually disregarded. Hence the rediscovery by the Platt Committee of a subject that had in fact been firmly in the syllabus (if not in the classroom) for the previous seven years.

Training in understanding and meeting the emotional needs of small children is still severely hindered by lack of conviction at the top levels of nursing. This can be seen in trends since the Platt Report of 1959. The topic of emotional needs is if anything handled with less emphasis rather than more. In 1964 the General Nursing Council issued a new 'Experimental' Syllabus of Subjects for Examination for the Nursing of Sick Children which continues in use (73, 74). Reference to the psychological development of children and the place of the family is extended, but in an outline form that deprives tutor and student of the stimulus of the evocative detail of the 1952 syllabus. For instance; compare the following with the excerpt on page 119 above:

> 'The basis of mental health; environment and constitution as a determinant of human behaviour. Family relationship and security. The importance of play. Social development during infancy, in pre-school years, at school. . . .'

There is no disputing that the 1952 syllabus was a much better guide to the basic considerations than is the bland outline of the 1964 syllabus. The rationale offered for the simplification was that it was necessary to make the 'Psychology for Nursing' section consistent with the sections dealing with diseases and physical care because 'knowledge changes'; and that a more detailed syllabus could go quickly out of date (72).

Bearing in mind the nature of the unawareness and resistances that operate (100, 101), it is probably also significant that, despite the emphases of the Platt Report, the word 'mother' no longer appears in the syllabus. Nor do the concepts of 'security in the mother–child relationship' or 'effects of separation from the mother'. The topic of mother and child, made vivid in the 1952 syllabus, is neutralized in the current syllabus.

It is surely also significant that the current syllabus does not mention the admission of mothers to hospital, though this was a main recommendation of Platt. Ten years after Platt, nurse training is based upon a syllabus that stops short at '*Visiting* children in hospital by parents and others'.

Another justification given for omitting the detail of the 1952 syllabus is that the tutor is thus freed from the constraint of a prescribed schema, and can determine the content that best suits her situation. This latitude might be warranted if nurse tutors had a sound basic training in child development, and were thus able to apply competent judgements to the content of their psychological teaching. But nurse tutors do not have this basic training in the psychological aspects of care.

Nurse tutors are trained in traditional nursing subjects related primarily to *the Causation, Nature, and Prevention of Disease*, but are given little more than a bird's-eye view of the wide field of individual, social, and group psychology. Within this scant coverage the emotional development and needs of young children has a minute place.[1]

Yet the Sister–Tutor's Diploma is deemed to qualify the holder to teach on all aspects of nursing, including the paediatric. She may have no previous experience of paediatric nursing other than eight weeks on a children's ward during general training as a State Registered Nurse (S.R.N.), yet on the basis of the Diploma be appointed

---

[1] The Sister–Tutor's Diploma is based upon a two-year full-time Extra-Mural Course provided by the General Nursing Council in association with the University of London (76). The syllabus sets out 485 hours of instruction and 360 hours of practice teaching. The traditional subjects of *Biology* (50 hours), *Physics and Chemistry* (75 hours), *Normal Structure and Function* (150 hours), *the Causation, Nature, and Prevention of Disease* (125 hours), *Development and Organization of the School of Nursing* (25 hours plus visits), and *the Practice of Education* (30 hours of lectures and 360 hours of practice teaching) are dealt with in depth. But *Psychology* is covered in 30 hours, and since the curriculum ranges widely over social relationships within the hospital, human development from infancy, mental health and the teacher, social and group psychology, learning theory, intelligence, etc., etc., the treatment can only be superficial.

The Final Examination for the Diploma is searching, but *Psychology* is not included and none of the questions set touch upon the emotional development and needs of young children (77).

sister-tutor in one of our leading children's hospitals. Such appointments are not uncommon (56).

This reflects a common misconception (perpetuated in a major policy statement of the Royal College of Nursing, see above, page 131) that the care of sick young children is not essentially different from that of sick adults. *It fails to recognize that by reason of their immaturity young children are distinctive and vulnerable, and that the quality of early experience affects their later social and emotional development.*

The present 'all-purpose' Sister–Tutor's Diploma does not provide an adequate basis for teaching the total care of child patients. It is therefore unsatisfactory to leave tutors to find their own way more or less unaided through the child development literature and without the necessary training to determine for themselves at what level the concepts will be taught. The understanding of emotional needs and the safeguarding of mental health is a complex area of knowledge and practice that cannot be entered into efficiently unless the tutors are themselves suitably taught, and unless they gain sufficient insight to accept the importance of mental health considerations.

It is therefore necessary either to increase substantially the psychological component in the syllabus or, more suitably, to offer the Diploma in alternative forms. Those wishing to specialize in paediatric nurse teaching would be taught and examined in depth on the social and emotional development of children and be awarded a Diploma whose title conveyed their special understanding of both the physical and emotional care of children. This might be a longer course than for the present Diploma and in recognition of this and of their contribution to preventive mental health these specialist tutors might be specially rewarded in their salary scales.

But indications are that in 1970 the General Nursing Council, like the paediatricians, regard the psychology of childhood as a non-priority subject which, like good manners, can be spread by encouragement and gentle persuasion. There are no relevant courses for tutors, as would be necessary if these were to treat the subject seriously; there are no recommendations about textbooks and other teaching aids—on the ground that it is not the function of the Council to press for conformity or to seem to direct tutors in what or how they teach. Bearing in mind how explicit the Council is about what must be taught on physical nursing, and how standards are enforced through the examination system, the difference in emphasis on the psychological aspects confirms the poor status of the subject.

The only direct influence brought to bear upon nursing schools is the gentle encouragement of inspectors during their infrequent visits. This comment implies no criticism of the inspectorate, who impress by their insight and by their concern that standards should improve until total care of the child is everywhere taught and practised; but the context within which they work is quite inappropriate for serious achievement in this area of training. That the context is so unrealistic ten years after Platt is still further confirmation that the matter is not perceived by the General Nursing Council to be one of urgency. Mental health is not a reality.

In England and Wales there are 1,030 training schools for the Nursing Register, of which 20 train for 'the part of the Register of Sick Children's Nurses'. In 1970 the Education Department[1] of the General Nursing Council

[1] With responsibility for all matters relating to the training of student and pupil nurses in general, children's, mental, and mental-subnormality nursing.

comprised 1 education officer, 2 assistant education officers, and 14 inspectors. Of these, 4 inspectors are on the Register of Mental Nursing, 8 on the General Register, and 2 on the Register of Sick Children's Nurses. This small band of inspectors have the heavy task of visiting hospitals, making reports on training to the General Nursing Council, advising the Council on nurse training and examinations, and advising the Council on trends that may necessitate changes in nurse training.

There are about 800 hospitals that admit children. The two Paediatric Inspectors always inspect the 20 children's hospitals, but can do no more than assist in the inspection of nurse training schools in general hospitals. Therefore not all of the 800 hospitals that admit children are visited by paediatric inspectors.

During their visits the inspectors deal with the whole range of paediatric nursing, and major emphasis is understandably given to those aspects which relate to physical care—the aspects which also dominate the examination papers. The most concerned of paediatric inspectors can do little more than offer suggestions about the teaching of emotional needs, being inhibited by the general orientation that this is a nontechnical subject —and by the fact that pass or failure in examinations is not involved.

Routine inspections are carried out every five years, more often when a new school is being established. This may be adequate for the supervision of traditional medico-nursing subjects of disease and disability, but cannot do much to promote psychological teaching. An anticipated increase in the inspectorate should enable inspections to be made every two years, but with the prevailing attitude to psychology this promises little improvement.

Young Children in Hospital

The examination papers set by the General Nursing Council confirm this relative inertia. In 1969 there were three sittings for the 'Final Examination of the Part of the Register for Sick Children's Nurses'[1]—each examination consisted of fourteen questions on 'All Aspects of the Care and Treatment of Sick Children' (75). In the February examination there was no question about the psychology of young children, though there was a question on the nursing of adolescents; in June the candidate was exceptionally invited to 'Discuss the part played by the mother in the care of her child while in hospital'; and in October the one question in the area of psychological understanding was 'Discuss the role of the nurse in the care of the sick child'.

But as only ten of the fourteen questions had to be answered, and none was compulsory, the Final State Examinations of February, June, and October 1969 could have been taken successfully without the candidate's having given evidence of understanding the emotional needs of young patients.

Examination papers indicate the level of knowledge and the orientation required for entry into a profession, and they give some indication of the assumptions within that profession. That it is possible to be admitted to the specialized Sick Children's Register without giving proof of psychological understanding confirms once more that this is not regarded as of high importance by those who determine the content of training. Otherwise, while recognizing that a good level of psychological teaching

[1] For those who wish to specialize in the nursing of sick children, and who (*a*) have been for 3 years in a children's hospital; or (*b*) after qualification as State Registered Nurses have been for 13 or 18 months in a children's hospital; or (*c*) have undertaken the Integrated Scheme of Training, which is based on a general hospital and a children's hospital and contains at least 15 months' experience with sick children.

cannot be obtained quickly from tutors of all ages and degrees of competence, the General Nursing Council might be expected to use the examination papers each year as a lever for gradually establishing higher and still higher levels of response from both tutors and nurses. Some tentative move in that direction is perhaps implied by the optional questions instanced from the 1969 examinations. But at the very least it could reasonably be expected that ten years after Platt, and seventeen years after the 1952 syllabus, the final examination for sick children's nurses would contain one or more obligatory questions on the psychological development and emotional needs of young children; that some explicit attention would be paid to mental health as well as to physical disease.

As at present constituted by Act of Parliament, the General Nursing Council is a body that inevitably reflects traditional nursing attitudes and concerns. There are 40 members, of whom 22 are nurses elected from the regions; of the 18 nominated by the Minister of Health and other departments of Government, the majority are required to be nurses, doctors, and hospital administrators; there are only two nominated places for which professions are not specified.

No specific provision is made for representation of the dynamic viewpoint that would be necessary if the importance of good and improving psychological teaching were to be constantly borne in mind. Only one place is reserved for the election of a paediatric nurse, which when set against the large number of nurses from psychiatry, subnormality, and all the other specialities indicates how minute is the claim of the most vulnerable patient of all—the young child. And, of course, with nurse training as it is, there is no guarantee that the single representative of paediatric nursing will have the dynamic viewpoint that is needed.

The constitution of this statutory body is currently under review. This would give an opportunity to ensure that psychological knowledge and conviction of the emotional needs of young patients is adequately built into the Council, its Education and Syllabus Committees, and the inspectorate. Within the existing constitution, and as a gesture of intent, the places that are not tied to named professions could be used to nominate two people from the mental health professions.

(ii) *The Royal College of Nursing.* There are two principal professional associations for State Registered Nurses— *The Royal College of Nursing* and *The Association of British Paediatric Nurses.* The R.C.N. is much the larger and represents in effect all registered nurses with the exception of a proportion of those on the Sick Children's Register who choose to remain outside the main body as members of the A.B.P.N.

The main purposes of The Royal College of Nursing include:

'To promote the science and art of nursing and the better education and training of nurses and their efficiency in the profession of nursing; to promote the advance of nursing as a profession in all or any of its branches. . . .'

In a memorandum submitted to the Platt Committee in 1957, the College said unambiguously that 'The first principle of mental health—to safeguard the mother–child relationship in the early years—should apply in hospital as elsewhere' and that 'Since the welfare of children in hospital depends to a large extent on the standard of nursing care it is essential that the *nurse must be adequately prepared and trained* [R.C.N.'s italics], not only in the required technical skills, but also in understanding the child's human needs'. It went on to advocate the admission of mothers as 'the surest way of safeguarding instinctive needs', unrestricted visiting, and patient assignment as the best form of nursing to meet the child's need of individual care by preventing the fragmentation of care that otherwise occurs (128). But, as with the paediatricians, there is no mention of the problem of deprivation of mothering care in long-stay children.

Having stated the considerations so cogently, it might have been expected that the Royal College of Nursing would have responded with urgency to the Platt Report's recommendations and implied criticisms of contemporary nursing practice. There could have been a series of national and local conferences, and an ongoing programme of seminars to promote the concepts and to examine the practical problems. But although the College specializes in further education, and organizes many conferences and study days, none has been devoted to the Platt Report of 1959.

There has been no sustained pressure by the College on its members to bring practice into line with the practical recommendations of Platt, no investigation of the practicability of patient assignment, no real sign of understanding that much of contemporary nursing practice constitutes an avoidable threat to the emotional well-being of young patients.

It appears that, as with the British Paediatric Association, understanding and concern lay with those who formulated the memorandum to Platt but did not in fact reflect the attitudes at the College. There was therefore no short-term action to remove avoidable stresses on young patients caused by out-dated systems of nursing.

The policy of the College on nursing education is contained in a 1964 Report on *A Reform of Nursing Education* (129), which says

'The conclusion is inescapable that the present form of training fails to give the student an adequate understanding of human, social and psychological problems. . . .'

The Report draws attention to the enormous difficulty, still unresolved after thirty years of committee study, of educating student nurses who are depended upon for service; and in a closely reasoned statement puts forward a 'revolutionary' scheme under which the nurse student would be a *bona fide* student, supplementary to staffing needs, who throughout most of her training would give service to patients only in the context of her studies. Separating education from service is in the view of the College an essential prerequisite of a significantly higher level of training, at the end of which the registered nurse

'. . . would have an understanding of social, psychological and environmental influences which affect behaviour patterns; she would be able to communicate effectively with others and establish a therapeutic relationship with patients.'[1]

If this advance in nurse education is ultimately achieved (and it is subject to acceptance and possible modification

[1] In 1967 the Minister of Health rejected the proposal to separate education from service, considering that 'great improvements can be made within the general structure of nurse training' (105). The College, nevertheless, continues to press for schools of nursing to be outside the service structure. In March 1970 the Government, concerned about the grave national shortage of nurses, set up an independent committee to look into the future role and training of the nurse so that her scarce skills can be used to best advantage (114).

by the General Nursing Council, and to great problems
of financing) the physical and emotional care of all
patients, including young children, will be much improved. But in this forward-looking report of about
20,000 words, not more than 100 words refer directly to
paediatric nursing, and this extract is not reassuring:
'. . . the principles of paediatrics are those of general
nursing applied to a special age group . . .'

That formulation perpetuates the failure to understand
that the hospitalization of young children presents a
different order of problem because of their immaturity,
their primary need of a stable relationship with a warm
and responsive mother-figure, and the risks that hospitalization holds for their later mental health. It is essential
that the care of young patients should be conceptualized
quite distinctly from that of all other patients.

(iii) *The Association of British Paediatric Nurses.* The
Association of British Paediatric Nurses claims to represent an elite of nurses who are specially competent to
deal with children in hospital—namely nurses on the
Sick Children's Register—and presses that all nursing of
children in hospital should be done by nurses with that
qualification (65). It could therefore be expected that this
professional body would be fully committed to promoting
optimal care for young children in hospital and a high
standard of professional training in the physical and
emotional aspects of illness and care.

But the memorandum submitted to the Platt Committee by
the A.B.P.N. (65) has an archaic quality that reflects narrow
concerns and uninsightful attitudes of a kind that were common twenty years earlier, when emotional upsets in child patients were complacently attributed to faults in the child's
family rather than to the effects of illness and hospitalization:

'Emotional responses of a child should be noted by the Ward Sister and unfavourable reactions investigated by the Lady Almoner. These reactions may be due to unsettled home conditions. . . .'

There is no reference to the special problem of the young patient arising from his attachment to the mother and his emotional reactions to illness and pain (11, 51, 60, 69, 78, 115).

Nothing is said about the value of patient-assignment nursing, about the desirability of preventing separation by admitting the mother, or about the advantages of unrestricted visiting:

'Daily visiting whenever possible. In cases of difficult or special feeding the parent to be encouraged to come in and handle the child before discharge.'

It is nowhere considered whether the hospital situation and systems of care might be improved. The implication is that if there are problems they are vested in the patient and his family, and that it is they who need handling:

'If the doctor thinks that there is going to be special difficulty with either the mother or the child, to make a special sign on the card. . . .'

It is unlikely that the memorandum made any contribution to the work of the Platt Committee, and, since the publication of the Report in 1959, the A.B.P.N. has continued to function as if impervious to the recommendations for training und practice. The programmes of its meetings perpetuate traditional concern with disease, disability, and professional status.

The A.B.P.N. gives an unfortunate impression of a static body, a relic of other times, instead of the leader in paediatric nursing thought and practice that it might be. The A.B.P.N. would be more justified in claiming to represent the specialists in child nursing if it were promoting training and practice in accord with present-day psychological knowledge.

That this is not so is sad, but not unexpected. As has been shown, it is not necessary to give evidence of psychological understanding in order to pass the final examinations for the Sick Children's Register and to become eligible for membership of the A.B.P.N. It is not to disparage the kindness and good intentions of paediatric nurses to say that their Association can be little better than the examinations that give entry to it. But an A.B.P.N. which is primarily concerned with status and with discussions of the physical disorders of children cannot be looked to for the necessary reforms in nursing care.

This view does not neglect the fact that there are individual members whose ward practice gives example of what might be; or that there are individual paediatric tutors whose teaching is infinitely better than examinations require.

THE HOSPITAL MANAGEMENT COMMITTEES AND THE PLATT REPORT

'The responsibility of the lay member of the management committee is first and foremost to the patient, whose representative, in a sense, he is. The committee's function, therefore, can be regarded as properly discharged when it has made the best possible provision for the patient within the financial scope permitted to it' (135).

Control of British hospitals is vested in management

committees whose membership includes 75 per cent laymen charged with representing the patients' interests. But the parents of young children do not perceive lay members in this light, and do not turn to them for help as in other circumstances they would turn to a Borough Councillor or Member of Parliament.

The Government's 'Green Paper' on the proposed reconstruction of the National Health Service acknowledges that the method whereby ultimate selection of all members of Regional Hospital Boards and Boards of Governors is made by the Secretary of State, and the ultimate selection of all members of Hospital Management Committees is made by Regional Hospital Boards, has been criticized as undemocratic; and that members of Hospital Management Committees as 'agents of agents of the Secretary of State', have a particularly slender democratic basis (66).

Two serious consequences of this method of appointing Hospital Management Committees are:

(a) that the lay members are not known to the people they represent, since they are neither elected by nor answerable to the local community;

(b) that, however worthy the lay members may be in other respects, their appointments tend to reflect local politics instead of relevant knowledge, experience, and concerns.

In 1969 the Cabinet Minister then concerned with finding ways to achieve greater participation by the community in this and other matters confirmed the view that many of the lay members who nominally 'manage' hospitals are not aware of patients' needs and whether they are, in fact, being met (79). In matters to do with the welfare of child patients lay members usually acquiesce in whatever forms of care are set by their medical and nursing officers—whether progressive or reactionary. In relation to the Platt Report, the Hospital Management Committees have been the least responsive of all. Hence the emergence of pressure groups such as N.A.W.C.H.

It is ironical that, in the first phase of a democratic society's attempt to humanize its hospitals, the system of unrepresentative appointment has been an obtuse barrier to the implementation of the Government's own en-lightened policies as set out in the Platt Report. However, early in 1970, the Secretary of State for Health and Social Security appointed four members of N.A.W.C.H. to Regional Hospital Boards and the Boards of Governors of teaching hospitals. This is understood to be the beginning of a new policy (in line with the Green Paper) to obtain more effective community representation and participation.

WHAT NEXT?

'Whereas the child, by reason of his physical and mental immaturity, needs special safeguards and care, the child of tender years shall not, save in exceptional circumstances, be separated from his mother.'

UNITED NATIONS, Declaration of the
Rights of the Child, 1959

'In 1966, the last year for which statistics are available, there were in England and Wales 374,000 admissions to hospital of children under five years of age.'

*Report on Hospital Inpatient Enquiry
for the Year* 1966 (106)

This is indeed a sobering picture for anyone hopeful of quick solutions to the plight of young patients. What is lacking in the professional entities upon which hospital practice depends is competence to apprehend the reality and urgency of mental health considerations in relation to young children with the result that (whatever may happen in the long term) short-term action is missing.

But despite this limitation of the professional bodies, the field situation has improved. Undoubtedly, the hospital professions are in varying degrees more sympathetic to the problems than they were ten years ago. Doctors and nurses are also parents and citizens, and as such they read the same newspapers and see the same television programmes as other citizens. So they have to some extent moved with the trend in community feeling about young children in hospital.

In many hospitals restrictive attitudes (though much less restrictive than ten years ago) persist and are reinforced by teaching that is insufficiently informed by modern knowledge about the emotional needs of young children. But there are a number of hospitals where tutors now teach in dynamic and relevant ways to which student nurses respond with the empathy and understanding that young people are ready to show when given the opportunity—that is, when their natural perceptions are encouraged instead of being crushed by the need to conform to unenlightened ward practices. Nurse tutors have also produced textbooks that, on the psychological side, deal unequivocally with the mother–child bond and its implications for unrestricted visiting and the admission of mothers (57, 67).

In this respect there is probably much more movement in nurse training than in medical training. A measure of this is that the author's films, *A Two-Year-Old Goes to Hospital*, 1952 (6) and *Going to Hospital With Mother*, 1958 (10), are now regular 'texts' for a number of nurse tutors. But these films are rarely used in medical schools, and when they are it is usually outside formal teaching and on the initiative of student societies.

Some nursing tutors are now using also the film studies of healthy young children, *Kate* (122, 125), *Jane* (123, 126), and *John* (124, 127) to illustrate normal development in accord with Platt recommendations, and to add to their students' understanding of psychological stress by showing the responses of young children to separation from the mother in different kinds of care and when illness and pain are absent.

When tutors of this quality are associated with wards that have accommodation for mothers and/or unrestricted visiting, there is the optimal situation in which theory and practice are in accord. But, particularly in some of the larger children's hospitals which attract top-level tutors and the cream of students, there can be serious frustrations for both tutors and students. Ward practice may conflict with mental health teaching. For instance, students taught the importance of relationships, including the function of substitute mothering, may find that in the wards they are actively discouraged from relating to the young patients. It is well known that teaching hospitals have been slower than some small general hospitals to follow Platt, perhaps because of their more complex structures and multiplicity of part-time consultants. Furthermore, even where psychological understanding is good, nursing systems that are top-heavy with students militate against the provision of stable nursing for unaccompanied young patients.

There has nevertheless been this random flowering of insightful paediatric nurse tutoring—spontaneous, and deriving from the tutor's personality, intelligence, and initiative (136). It is noticeable that in a large children's hospital, where student nurses spend three years and the aspiring paediatrician perhaps no more than six months, the psychological understanding of the young nurses may be infinitely and embarrassingly greater than that of the young medicals.

But the achievements of these individual nurse tutors highlight the failure of the professional associations— the British Paediatric Association, the General Nursing Council, the Royal College of Nursing, and the Association of British Paediatric Nurses—to meet the Platt Report's call to bring about early improvement in the training of medical and nursing students.

The dilemma of the professions caring for young children in hospital is that, at a point where movement into psychological understanding is needed, many of the leaders are blinkered by years of non-psychological working and thinking. They are unaware of the limits of their knowledge.

What is now needed is a Government Commission to make a full and comprehensive technical appraisal of the provisions for the care of children in hospital. Whatever the lay representation thereon, the Commission would consist essentially of experts drawn from all relevant branches of knowledge. In order to ensure that due attention was paid to the disciplines concerned with mental health, there would be an independent chairman.

The Commission would have immediate benefit of work already done on the future of medical and nursing training, but not yet implemented—the report of the Royal Commission on Medical Education, 1968 (130) and the report of the Royal College of Nursing, 1964, *A Reform of Nurse Training* (129). Both reports urge the need for integrated trainings that give due weight to physical, psychological, and sociological factors. One explicit *raison d'être* for the Commission would be recognition of the need to safeguard the mental health of young patients, and it would be understood that the representatives of the psychological disciplines had important and valid contributions to make.

The Commission would have ample resources of time and money in order to investigate the practical and technical considerations involved in achieving integrated training of professional staff and optimal care for child patients. The scope and complexity of an inquiry intended to have practical outcome would be great, ranging over all aspects of medicine and surgery, nursing, psychology, and administration.

The Commission might be set up on a semi-permanent or long-term basis, and have the means to initiate prototype care and teaching units in order to investigate the requirements of total care (medical and psychological) together with good medical and nursing training.

On this basis the Commission would publish a series of practical reports and also have open for inspection its working prototypes—through which, incidentally, would pass young doctors and nurses who would carry into other settings their trainings in integrated total care.

Based somewhat on the precedent of the Curtis Committee which investigated the institutional care of healthy children (13) the principal report(s) of the Commission would provide the bases for certain legislation to obtain agreed standards of training and provision. It was a weakness of the Children Act, 1948, upon which the care of healthy children in institutions and the training of staff is based, that it did not legislate for children and staff in hospitals. Twenty years later it is time to do so. The basic needs of young children in hospitals and other institutions are in many ways similar.

Young Children in Hospital

We are fortunate that in Britain the problems of caring for young children in hospital are so freely discussed. Although there is discontent, this does not mean that in other countries the situation is better.

The opposite is true.

On the Continent of Europe there is little or no public discussion of young children in hospitals. This is not because all is well, but because the problem has not yet broken through to public concern. In much of France, Germany, Holland, Belgium, Spain, Denmark, Italy, Austria, and elsewhere restrictions on access to child patients are as severe as they were in Britain twenty or thirty years ago, and unrestricted visiting and the accommodation of mothers would rarely be regarded as for serious discussion. In Eastern Europe the situation is at least as restrictive.

In the United States, the quality of care is often determined by how much the parents can afford to pay. There are some paediatric wards with exceptional facilities, but many others where conditions are more depriving than any to be found in Britain. Furthermore, in the United States the gap between the hospital professions and the community is generally wide. There is no movement comparable to N.A.W.C.H. in which parents and professionals meet to consider matters of mutual concern.

There is no other country in the world where the interchange between the community and the hospital professions is as free as in Britain, where bridges have been built between hospitals and community as has happened in this country during the past twenty years.

Our discontents are a sign of progress. This positive aspect has to be borne in mind as the debates and pressures continue—that these are the phenomena of a concerned democratic society, and not of one that lags behind any other.

The changes in training and administration that are necessary to obtain optimal child-patient care will probably be achieved in time. But this will be a long time, and vicissitudes could intervene to delay or distort objectives. Therefore the need continues for vigilance and an informed public opinion.

While the professions and administrations come slowly to terms with the problems of young patients, the best safeguard the community can provide is to open up hospitals to parents—and at the same time to educate parents about the meaning of hospitalization to their children and what they can do to help. This educational work could appropriately be undertaken by N.A.W.C.H. if it had the resources.

N.A.W.C.H. has not only worked effectively to keep alive the Platt Report. It has done a rare service in showing how lay and professional people can work together. Well ahead of the Green Paper, N.A.W.C.H. has helped to create the climate within which the proposals for community participation in running the Health Service are most likely to succeed.

Successive Ministers have acknowledged the value of its work. But N.A.W.C.H. is a voluntary body, working on a shoestring. The movement must be adequately financed if it is to survive and expand the work in the many ways that are needed.

It is in the British tradition that a new area of social concern should be developed by inspired volunteers, and at an appropriate point be financed and stabilized. That time has now come for N.A.W.C.H., an organization of proven efficiency and concern in promoting the implementation of the Ministry's enlightened policies on the welfare of children in hospital.

REFERENCES

1. BOWLBY, J. (1951) *Maternal Care and Mental Health*. World Health Organization Monograph Series, No. 2, Geneva. (U.K., H.M.S.O.; U.S.A., Columbia Univ. Press.) Abridged version of above: *Child Care and the Growth of Love*. Harmondsworth: Pelican Books A271 (1953).

2. BOWLBY, J. (1958) 'Separation of Mother and Child.' (A Letter) *Lancet*, March 1, 480.

3. BOWLBY, J., AINSWORTH, M., BOSTON, M., and ROSENBLUTH, D. (1956) 'The Effects of Mother-Child Separation: A Follow-up Study.' *Brit. J. med. Psychol.* 3 and 4, 211–47.

4. BOWLBY, J., ROBERTSON, J., and ROSENBLUTH, D. (1952). 'A Two-Year-Old Goes to Hospital.' *Psychoanal. Study Child*, 7, 82–94.

5. ROBERTSON, J., and BOWLBY, J. (1952) 'Recent Trends in Care of Deprived Children in the U.K.' *Bulletin of the World Federation for Mental Health*, Vol. 4, No. 3.

6. ROBERTSON, J. (1953a) Film: *A Two-Year-Old Goes to Hospital*. 16mm. Snd. 45 minutes. English or French. London: Tavistock Clinic; New York University Film Library.

7. ROBERTSON, J. (1953b) Guide to the film *A Two-Year-Old Goes to Hospital*. London: Tavistock Publications.

8. ROBERTSON, J. (1953c) 'Some Responses of Young Children to Loss of Maternal Care.' *Nursing Times*, April, 382–6. 'L'Attitude de jeunes enfants privés de soins maternels.' *L'Infirmière*, Belgique, 31, No. 4–6.

9. ROBERTSON, J. (1955) 'Young Children in Long-Term Hospitals.' *Nursing Times*, 23 Sept.

10. ROBERTSON, J. (1958) Film: *Going to Hospital with*

Mother. 16mm. Snd. 45 minutes. London: Tavistock Institute of Human Relations; New York University Film Library.

11. ROBERTSON, JOYCE (1956) 'A Mother's Observations on the Tonsillectomy of Her Four-Year-Old Daughter.' With Comments by Anna Freud. *Psychoanal. Study Child*, 11, 410-27; *Nursing Times*, 15 Nov., 1957, 1395-407.

12. BURLINGHAM, D., and FREUD, A. (1942) *Young Children in Wartime*. (Report of a residential war nursery.) London: Allen and Unwin.

13. CARE OF CHILDREN COMMITTEE (1946) *Report . . . presented by the Secretary of State for the Home Department, the Minister of Health and the Minister of Education*. (Curtis Report) London: H.M.S.O.

14. CENTRAL COUNCIL FOR HEALTH EDUCATION (1957) *Coming Into Hospital*. A Leaflet. London.

15. CHILD DEVELOPMENT CENTER (1953) *Going to the Hospital*. Children's Hospital of the East Bay, Oakland, California.

16. CRAIG, J., and MCKAY, E. (1958) 'Working of a Mother and Baby Unit.' *Brit. med. J.* 1, 275-7.

17. EDELSTON, H. (1943) 'Separation Anxiety in Young Children: Study of Hospital Cases.' *Genet. Psychol. Monogr.*, 28, 3-95.

18. FAIRFIELD HOSPITAL (1953) *Report of Board of Management*. Also personal communication from the Medical Superintendent.

19. FAUST, O. A. (1952) 'Reducing Emotional Trauma in Hospitalized Children: A Study in Psychosomatic Pediatrics,' in *Reducing Emotional Trauma in Hospitalized Children*, a report by Departments of Pediatrics and Anesthesiology, Albany Medical College, Albany, N.Y.

20. FRANK, R. (1952) 'Parents and the Pediatric Nurse.' *Amer. J. Nursing*, 52, 76-77.

21. FREUD, A. (1953) 'Film Review: A Two-Year-

Old Goes to Hospital.' *Psychoanal. Study Child*, 7, 82-94.

22. FREUD, A. (1957) See 11 above.

23. GODFREY, A. E. (1955) 'A Study of Nursing Care Designed to Assist Hospitalized Children and their Parents in their Separation.' *Nursing Research*, Vol. 4, No. 2, 52-69.

24. HARDEN, L. M. (1953) 'Child Care Centers Provide Experience for Students.' *Amer. J. Nursing*, Vol. 3, No. 1, 61-2.

25. HEMMENDINGER, M. (1956) 'Admit Parents at all Times.' *Child Study*, Vol. XXXIV, No. 1, 3-9.

26. HUNT, A.D., and TRUSSELL, R.E. (1955) 'They Let Parents Help in Children's Care.' *The Modern Hospital*, Sept. (Also personal communication from Dr. Hunt, Director of Pediatric Services.)

27. ILLINGWORTH, R. S., and HOLT, K. S. (1955) 'Children in Hospital: Some Observations on their Reactions with Special Reference to Daily Visiting.' *Lancet*, 17 Dec., 1257-62.

28. INTERNATIONAL UNION FOR CHILD WELFARE (1955) Proceedings of the World Child Welfare Congress. 1954, Geneva: I.U.C.W.

29. JACKSON, E. B. (1942) 'Treatment of the Young Child in the Hospital.' *Amer. J. Orthopsychiatr.* 12, 56-67.

30. JACOB, C. G. (1953) 'A Study of the Young Child's Contacts with Staff Members in a Selected Pediatric Hospital.' *Nursing Research*, June, 2, 1.

31. JACOBS, J. J. M. (1957) 'Anxiety and Self-Reproach in Parents.' *Medical Press*, 8 May.

32. JESSNER, L., and KAPLAN, S. (1949) 'Observations on the Emotional Reactions of Children to Tonsillectomy and Adenoidectomy.' In Transactions of the Third Conference on *Problems of Infancy and Childhood*, edited by M. J. E. Senn. New York: Josiah Macy, Jr. Foundation.

33. LANCET (1949) 'Children in Hospital. A Discussion.' May 7, 784-6.

34. LANCET (1949) 'Disabilities No. 31: Hospitalization in Childhood.' 4 June, 975-6.

35. LEVY, D. (1945) 'Psychic Trauma of Operations in Children . . .' *Amer. J. Dis. Child.*, 69, 7-25.

36. LIGHTWOOD, R., *et al.* (1957) 'Home Care for Sick Children.' *Lancet*, 9 Feb., 313-17.

37. MACCARTHY, D. (1957) 'Mothers in a Children's Ward.' *Public Health*, October.

38. MAC KEITH, R. (1953) 'Children in Hospital: Preparation for Operation.' *Lancet*, 2, 843-5.

39. MATIC, V. (1957) 'A Hospital Without Nurses.' *Bulletin of the World Federation for Mental Health*, August.

40. MORGAN, M. L., and LLOYD, B. J. (1955) 'Parents Invited, a: The Mother's View; b: The Nurse's View.' *Nursing Outlook*, May, 256-9.

41. NURSING TIMES (1957) 'The Mind of a Young Child.' (Editorial) 15 Nov., 1289-90.

42. PICKERILL, C. M., and PICKERILL, H. P. (1946) 'Keeping Mother and Baby Together.' *Brit. med. J.*, 2, 337.

43. POWERS, G. F. (1948) 'Humanizing Hospital Experiences.' *Amer. J. Dis. Child*, 76, 365-79.

44. PRUGH, D. G., *et al.* (1953) 'A Study of the Emotional Reactions of Children and Families to Hospitalization and Illness.' *Amer. J. Orthopsychiat.* 23, 70-106.

45. SHARP, J. (1950) 'Nursing By Case Assignment.' *Nursing Times*, 46, 4-6.

46. SPENCE, J. C. (1946) *The Purpose of the Family: A Guide to the Care of Children.* London: Epworth Press.

47. SPENCE, J. C. (1947) 'Care of Children in Hospital.' *Brit. med. J.*, 1, 125-30.

48. SPENCE, J. C. (1951) 'The Doctor, The Nurse, and the Sick Child.' *Amer. J. Nursing*, 51, No. 1.

49. STEVENS, M. (1949) 'Visitors are Welcome in the Pediatric Ward.' *Amer. J. Nursing,* 49, 233-5.

50. VAUGHAN, G. F. (1957) 'Children in Hospital.' *Lancet,* June 1, 1117-20.

51. WALLACE, M., and FEINAUER, V. (1948) 'Understanding a Sick Child's Behaviour.' *Amer. J. Nursing,* 48, 517-22.

52. WILSON, A. T. M. (1950) *Hospital Nursing Auxiliaries.* London: Tavistock Publications.

53. WINKLEY, R. (1952) 'Case Worker's Participation in Preparation for Tonsillectomy in Children.' *Report of Albany Research Project*—see FAUST above.

54. WINNICOTT, D. W. (1948) 'Paediatrics and Psychiatry.' In *Collected Papers: through Paediatrics to Psycho-Analysis.* London: Tavistock Publications, 1958.

55. WINNICOTT, D. W. (1953) 'Transitional Objects and Transitional Phenomena.' In *Collected Papers: through Paediatrics to Psycho-Analysis.* London: Tavistock Publications, 1958.

REFERENCES TO POSTSCRIPT 1970

56. ADVERTISEMENT (1970) A New Post for Senior Nursing Officer, Teaching Grade 8 (Responsible for 2 intakes of the 3-year 8-month Scheme for S.R.N./R.S.C.N.). Qualifications: Experienced Tutor S.R.N. or S.R.N. & R.S.C.N. *Nursing Mirror,* 13 February, p. 88.

57. ALTSCHUL, A. (1965) *Psychology for Nurses.* London: Baillière, Tindall & Cassell.

58. BENDALL, E., and RAYBOULD, E. (1969) *A History of the General Nursing Council for England and Wales.* London: Lewis.

59. BERGMAN, A. B., SHRAND, H., and OPPE, T. E. (1965) 'A Pediatric Home Care Program in London —10 Years Experience.' *Pediatr.* 36, 314-321.

60. BERGMAN, T. (1965) *Children in the Hospital.* New York: International Universities Press.

61. BENIAN, R. C. (1970) 'Children with Burns.' *Maternal and Child Care*, 6, 57, 215-224.

62. BLAKE, F. G., WRIGHT, F. H., and WAECHTER, E. (1970) *Nursing Care of Children*. Philadelphia: Lippincott.

63. BRAIN, D. J., and MACLAY, INGE (1968) 'Controlled Study of Mothers and Children in Hospital.' *Brit. med. J.*, 2, 278-280.

64. BRITISH PAEDIATRIC ASSOCIATION (1959) 'The Welfare of Children in Hospital.' *Lancet*, 1, 166-9.

65. BRITISH PAEDIATRIC NURSES, ASSOCIATION OF (1957) *Arrangements in Hospital for the Welfare of Ill Children* (Unpublished Memorandum to the Platt Committee).

66. DEPARTMENT OF HEALTH AND SOCIAL SECURITY (1970) *The Future Structure of the National Health Service*. London: H.M.S.O.

67. DUNCOMBE, A. A., and WELLER, B. (1969) *Paediatric Nursing*. London: Baillière, Tindall & Cassell.

68. FAGIN, C. M. (1966) *The Effects of Maternal Attendance during Hospitalization on the Post Hospital Behaviour of Young Children: A Comparative Study*. Philadelphia: F. A. Davis.

69. FREUD, A. (1952) 'The Role of Bodily Illness in the Mental Life of Children.' *Psychoanal. Study Child*, 7, 69-81.

70. FREUD, A. (1970) Film Review: *John, aged 17 months, For Nine Days in a Residential Nursery*. *Psychoanal. Study Child*, 24.

71. GENERAL NURSING COUNCIL (1952a) *Syllabus of Subjects for Examination for the Certificate of Nursing Sick Children*. London: General Nursing Council.

72. GENERAL NURSING COUNCIL (1952b) *Guide to the Syllabus of Examination for the Part of the Register for Sick Children's Nurses*. London: General Nursing Council.

73. GENERAL NURSING COUNCIL (1964a) *Syllabus of Subjects for Examination for the Certificate of the Nursing of Sick Children*. London: General Nursing Council.

74. GENERAL NURSING COUNCIL (1964b) *Guide to the Syllabus of Subjects for Examination for the Certificate of the Nursing of Sick Children*. London: General Nursing Council.

75. GENERAL NURSING COUNCIL (1969a) *Final State Examination for the Part of the Register for Sick Children's Nurses. (All Aspects of the Care and Treatment of Sick Children)*. February, June, and October. London: General Nursing Council.

76. GENERAL NURSING COUNCIL (1969b) *Regulations for the Sister-Tutor's Diploma*. University of London.

77. GENERAL NURSING COUNCIL (1969c) *Examination Papers for the Sister Tutor's Diploma*, 1969. University of London.

78. GORDON, B. (1969) 'Studying Child Reactions to Life in the Hospital.' *Maternal and Child Care*, 5, 48.

79. HART, J. (1969) 'Mothers Won in Clash with Hospitals.' London: *The Times*, 20 September.

79a. HOPKINS, J. (1969) 'Children in Hospital. Observations on the Reactions of Chinese Children to Hospitalization with Implications for Child Care Practices.' *Far East med. J.*, 5, Sept., 279-84.

80. HUBBLE, D. V., JACKSON, A. D. M., and ELLIS, J. R. (1969) 'A Symposium on the Past, Present, and Future of British Paediatrics.' *Brit. J. med. Educ.*, 3, 256-7.

81. JACKSON, A. D. M. (1966) 'A Survey of Paediatric Teaching in The Undergraduate Medical Schools of the United Kingdom.' *Brit. J. med. Educ.*, 1, 25-39.

82. JACOBY, N. M. (1969) 'Unrestricted Visiting in a Children's Ward. The First Twenty Years.' *Lancet*, 2, 584-586.

83. JAMES, V. J., Jr., and WHEELER, W. E. (1969) 'The Care-By-Patient Unit.' *Pediatr.* 43, No. 4, Part 1, 488-494.

84. JOINT COMMITTEE: Institute of Child Health, Society of Medical Officers of Health, and Population Investigation Committee (1954) *An Account of Hospital Admissions in the Pre-School Period.* London: Institute of Child Health.

85. JOLLY, H. (1969) 'Pediatrics in Great Britain.' *Clinical Pediatr.* 8, No. 9, 540-2.

86. LAWRIE, R. (1964) 'Operating on Children as Day Cases.' *Lancet*, 2, 1289-1291.

87. LIPTON, S. D. (1962) 'On the Psychology of Childhood Tonsillectomy.' *Psychoanal. Study Child.*, 17.

88. LOOMIS, W. G. (1967) 'The Use of a Foster-Grandparent in the Psychotherapy of a Pre-School Child on a Pediatric Ward.' *Clinical Pediatrics*, 6, 384-386.

89. MACCARTHY, D. (1958) 'The Children's Unit at Amersham General Hospital.' In *Guide to the Film: Going to Hospital With Mother*, Robertson, J. London: Tavistock Institute of Human Relations.

90. MACCARTHY, D., LINDSAY, M., and MORRIS, I. (1962) 'Children in Hospital With Mothers.' *Lancet*, 1, 603-608.

91. MACCARTHY, D., and LOWENSTEIN, H. (1969) *Separations and Reunions. Film Studies I and II: Susan* (17 months) Emotional Convalescence After Cleft Palate Repair: and *Robert* (20 months) Salmonella Enteritis, 18 Days in Isolation Hospital. 16mm, Sound, 25 mins.
Film Studies III and IV: Vanessa (14 months) Gastro-enteritis, a brief hospitalization: and *Alicia* (15 months) Coeliac Disease, Significant Moments During Eight Hours of 24th Hospital Day. 16mm, Sound, 10 mins. (Both films should be seen together.)

Both above films from Concord Films Council, Nacton, Ipswich, Suffolk.

92. MACCARTHY, D., and MAC KEITH, R. C. (1965) 'A Parent's Voice.' *Lancet*, 18 Dec., 1289-91.

93. MACCARTHY, D., and MORRIS, I. (1959) 'Mother and Child in Hospital: The Practical Aspects.' *Nursing Times*, 55, 8, 219-222.

94. MAC KEITH, R. C. (1969) 'Empathy in the Hospital.' *Nursing Times*, 28 Aug.

95. MASON, E. A. (1962) Film: *Children in the Hospital*. 16mm, Sound, 44 minutes. Booklet. Chicago: International Film Bureau.

96. MASON, E. A. (1965) 'The Hospitalized Child: His Emotional Needs.' *New England J. Med.*, 272, 406-414.

97. MASON, E. A. (1967) 'Films on Children's Hospitalization and Maternal Deprivation: An Annotated Bibliography.' *Community Mental Health Journal*, 3, 4, 420-3.

98. MEADOW, S. R. (1964) ' "No, thanks, I'd rather stay at home". Mothers who do not want to accompany their children into hospital—their class, their families, and their reading habits.' *Brit. med. J.*, 2, 813.

99. MEADOW, S. R. (1969) 'The Captive Mother.' *Arch. Dis. Childh.* 44, 362-7.

100. MENZIES, E. P. (1960) *The Functioning of Social Systems as a Defence against Anxiety: A Study of the Nursing System of a General Hospital*. London: Tavistock Institute.

101. MENZIES, E. P. (1961) 'Nurses Under Stress.' *Nursing Times*, 57, 5, 6, 7.

102. MINISTRY OF HEALTH (Central Health Services Council) (1959) *The Welfare of Children in Hospital. Report of the Committee*. ('The Platt Report') London: H.M.S.O.

103. MINISTRY OF HEALTH (1964) *Hospital Building Note No. 23. Children's Ward*. London: H.M.S.O.

104. MINISTRY OF HEALTH (1964) *Sick Children (Accommodation for Mothers)*. Answer to a Question in the House of Commons. *Hansard*, 697, 1470. London: H.M.S.O.

105. MINISTRY OF HEALTH (1967) *Training of Nurses*. Memorandum M/R86/8D. London: Ministry of Health.

106. MINISTRY OF HEALTH AND GENERAL REGISTER OFFICE (1968) *Report on Hospital Inpatient Enquiry for the year 1966*. Part I, Tables. London: H.M.S.O.

107. MINISTRY OF HEALTH (1970) (See DEPARTMENT OF HEALTH AND SOCIAL SECURITY)

108. MORRIS, D. (1964) 'Mother Care for Children.' *Parents*, December.

109. N.A.W.C.H. (1967) *Hospital Admission Leaflet*. London: National Association for the Welfare of Children in Hospital.

110. N.A.W.C.H. (1969) *Visiting Hours for Sick Children in Hospital: A Survey*. London: National Association for the Welfare of Children in Hospital.

111. NOBLE, E. (1967) *Play With the Sick Child*. London: Faber.

112. NUFFIELD FOUNDATION (1963) *Children in Hospital: Studies in Planning*. Oxford University Press.

113. NURSING TIMES (1969) 'The Separated Child' (Review of film *John*). 65, 48, 27 November.

114. NURSING TIMES (1970) Editorial: 'Briggs's Task.' *Nursing Times*, 66, 10, 289.

115. PLANK, E. (1964) *Working With Children in Hospitals*. London: Tavistock Publications. New York: Western Reserve University Press.

116. RILEY, I. D. *et al.* (1965) 'Mother and Child in Hospital—Two Years' Experience.' *Brit. med. J.* 2, 990-992.

117. ROBERTSON, J. (1958a) Film: *Going to Hospital With Mother*. 16mm, Sound, 40 minutes. English or French

(A l'hôpital avec Maman) London: Tavistock Institute of Human Relations; New York University Film Library; and film libraries throughout the world.

118. ROBERTSON, J. (1958b) *Guide to the Film 'Going to Hospital With Mother'* (With an Appendix by Dr. Dermod MacCarthy). London: Tavistock Institute of Human Relations.

119. ROBERTSON, J. (1961) 'Children in Hospital.' London: *The Observer*, Jan. 15, 22, 29.

120. ROBERTSON, J. (1962) *Hospitals and Children: A Parent's-Eye View.* (Foreword by Sir Harry Platt, Bt.) London: Gollancz; New York: International Universities Press.

121. ROBERTSON, J. (1968) 'The Long-Stay Child in Hospital.' *Maternal and Child Care*, 4, 161-166.
ROBERTSON, J. and J. *Young Children in Brief Separation.* A series of films on the responses of young children of previous good experience to separation from the mother when the substitute care meets, or fails to meet, their emotional needs.

122. —— (1967) Film 1: *Kate: 2 years, 5 months. In Fostercare for 27 Days.* 16mm, Sound, 33 minutes.

123. —— (1968) Film 2: *Jane, 17 months, In Fostercare for 10 Days.* 16mm, Sound, 37 minutes.

124. —— (1969) Film 3: *John, 17 months, For Nine Days in a Residential Nursery.* 16mm, Sound, 45 minutes.

125. —— (1967) Guide to the film *Kate*, above.

126. —— (1968) Guide to the film *Jane*, above.

127. —— (1969) Guide to the film *John*, above.
London: Tavistock Institute of Human Relations; New York: New York University Film Library; and from film libraries elsewhere.

128. ROYAL COLLEGE OF NURSING (1957) *The Welfare of Children in Hospital* (Unpublished Memorandum). London: Royal College of Nursing.

129. ROYAL COLLEGE OF NURSING (1964) *A Reform*

of Children in Hospital (Unpublished Memorandum). London: Royal College of Nursing.

129. ROYAL COLLEGE OF NURSING (1964) *A Reform of Nurse Training: First Report of a Special Committee on Nurse Education*. London: Royal College of Nursing.

130. ROYAL COMMISSION ON MEDICAL EDUCATION (1968) *Report* (Todd Report). London: H.M.S.O.

131. SHORE, M. F. (Ed) (1967) *'Red is the Color of Hurting.' Planning for Children in the Hospital*. (Proceedings of a Workshop on Mental Health Planning for Pediatric Hospitals, New York 1965). Washington: U.S. Dept. of Health, Education, and Welfare; Public Health Service.

132. SHRAND, H. (1964) 'Home Care Scheme for Children.' *Nursing Times*, 60, 35, 1113-1116.

133. SHRAND, H. (1965) 'Behaviour Changes in Sick Children Nursed at Home.' *Pediatr*. 36, 604-607.

134. STARK, J. M. (1969) The American Foster-Grandparents Programme: A Service for Old People and Children.' *Social and Economic Administration*, 3, 3, 178-184.

135. STUART-CLARK, A. C. (1960) *Administering the Hospital Group: The Work of the Management Committee Member*. London: Institute of Hospital Administrators.

136. WELLER, B. F. (1969) 'Training Paediatric Nurses.' *Maternal and Child Care*, 5, 47, 54-6.

137. WINNICOTT, D. W. (1959) 'Film Review: Going to Hospital With Mother.' *Int. J. Psycho-Anal.*, 40, 1.

138. WOODWARD, J., and JACKSON, D. (1961) 'Emotional Reactions in Burned Children and Their Mothers.' *Brit. J. Plastic Surgery*, 13, 4, 316-324.

About the Author

JAMES ROBERTSON is a Scotsman. At one time a psychiatric social worker, he is now a psychoanalyst dividing his time between private practice and research. He is married and has two daughters.

He has for twenty years successfully combined the roles of scientist and propagandist. His research on the effects on young children of separation from the mother on admission to hospitals and other institutions has always had application in mind, and his writings and complementary films *A Two-Year-Old Goes to Hospital* and *Going to Hospital With Mother* have combined to influence the institutional care of young children in many parts of the world. Currently he and his wife Joyce Robertson, their daughters now being grown up, are working together on *Young Children in Brief Separation*. In this project they have taken a series of young children into their own home while the mothers are in hospital, to investigate in the interests of science what resources the children have for coping with loss of the mother when relieved of as many other stresses as possible; and on the practical side to discover how best fostercare might be given. The first publications are five films—*Jane*, *Lucy*, *Thomas* and *Kate* being studies of their four fosterchildren and *John* a harrowing contrast study of the deterioration of a 17-month-old child in a well-intentioned residential nursery that fails to meet his need of a mother-substitute.